FAQ

Alzheimer's Disease

FREQUENTLY ASKED QUESTIONS

Making Sense of the Journey

Also by Frena Gray-Davidson

The Alzheimer's Sourcebook for Caregivers:
A Practical Guide for Getting Through the Day

FAQ

Alzheimer's Disease

FREQUENTLY ASKED QUESTIONS

Making Sense of the Journey

by

Frena Gray-Davidson

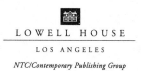

LOWELL HOUSE

LOS ANGELES

NTC/Contemporary Publishing Group

Library of Congress Cataloging in Publication Data

Gray-Davidson, Frena.
     Alzheimer's FAQ: frequently asked questions / by Frena Gray-Davidson.
         p.   cm.
     Includes bibliographical references and index.
     ISBN 0-7373-0079-5
     1. Alzheimer's disease—Miscellanea.   2. Alzheimer's disease—
Patients—Home care—Miscellanea. I. Title.
RC523.2.D377   1997
616.8'31—dc21   97-40587
                                               CIP

Published by Lowell House
A division of NTC/Contemporary Publishing Group, Inc.
4255 West Touhy Avenue, Lincolnwood, Illinois 60646-1975 U.S.A.

Copyright © 1998, 1999 by NTC/Contemporary Publishing Group.

Printed in the United States of America

International Standard Book Number: 0-7373-0079-5

00 01 02 03 04 DHD 18 17 16 15 14 13 12 11 10 9 8 7 6 5 4 3 2

To all caregivers

Contents

Acknowledgments

The questions in this book have come from three sources:

First, from the participants of my international workshops for family members and for professional care staff, in which I try to teach the basics of making meaningful relationships with people with Alzheimer's and similar dementias.

Second, from people who have logged on to my Web page on the Internet and accepted my invitation to e-mail me with questions.

And third, from readers of my first book on Alzheimer's, *The Alzheimer's Sourcebook*, who have written with their experiences and viewpoints.

I want to thank all these people and to honor every caregiver, whether helping a family member or working in a professional setting.

This great army of spiritual warriors, most of whom feel alone and unacknowledged, walk into the outer edges of the chaos we call Alzheimer's because they care and because they are needed.

May they all share any merit that comes from helping others understand what we do and why it matters.

Introduction

Alzheimer's caregiving has been a spiritual journey for me, and the people with Alzheimer's whom I cared for have been a daily blessing and my most respected teachers.

I've been fortunate in the sense that it was not family crisis that brought me into contact with Alzheimer's. As a caregiver, I found a home through Alzheimer's when I needed one. The happy synchronicity of an elderly woman in Berkeley, California, who needed one more person to care for her came at a time when I was desperately trying to figure out how to stay and work in the United States, the country of my choice. Since then I have been led on a rich and profoundly moving journey into my own spiritual awakening.

As a practicing Buddhist meditator, I had read plenty about compassion and living with loving-kindness. I experienced this during the fifteen colorful years I spent in Asia, where I was trying to find answers to mysteries within me and in the world around me. I was blessed by meeting many healers and meditators: Tibetan doctors in the Himalayas; sacred healers in the Hindu tradition who healed with prayer, herbs, and sacred ash; masked healers in Sri Lanka who used dance, ritual, and herbal ceremonies to drive out disease and demons. It was my good fortune to study Chinese medicine with a traditional Chinese healer as well as tai chi with a martial arts master. In the process I began to lose a little of my Western sense of rigidity.

I saw how often sacred life, healing, and medicine are woven into one rich cloth. Even in Hong Kong, where most visitors witness a modern urban lifestyle, mystics and healers from the Taoist tradition use divination, ritual, and sacred ceremony to help others. I experienced receiving chi energy from healers who could manipulate the chi of others without ever laying hands on them.

But in all my explorations—with meditation, the insights I received into healing, the ways in which I tried to develop my capacity to care and to live as a spiritually centered person—nothing has touched me as much as my work with people who have Alzheimer's disease.

That was another accidental meeting—or blessed synchronicity. When I began to realize that being on the outer edge of other societies was not enough, that I wanted to find a place that felt like home, I picked America—not the tired, jaded, rather whiny country of my birth, Britain, but the exuberant, get-up-and-go, optimistic, and somewhat brash cousin country, the United States.

I love the fact that it is a place where people can do anything they want to, where people achieve as much as they are capable of, and where everyone thinks they are as good as anyone else—and they're right. For all its difficulties—and I know them well—America is still the beautiful and the bright, especially in comparison to the many other societies I experienced.

I started out by doing the traditional work of a poor female immigrant: cleaning houses (and I hated to clean my own) and scrubbing floors on my knees. I took jobs in restaurants I wouldn't eat in if you paid me—pizza dives in Oakland—and did yardwork that consisted mainly of cleaning up after other people's dogs.

I often asked myself if giving up a thriving writing career in Hong Kong—where I had been well paid and had status, where everyone knew me, where I could choose my writing projects—was worth this struggle. When I prayed that somehow my life would deepen, that my heart would open and my spirit really wake up in some new way, I did not think one slightly plump German-accented seventy-nine-year-old Jewish intellectual would start the pathway for me.

I loved her from the beginning. She was the start of a line of sacred teachers who arrived in the shape of wild and dear old women, who thought their long-dead fathers were coming home to tea, who thought they were in Dresden or Paris but not the land of the free, and who wanted safety, love, and reassurance in a world gone crazy. These women made sense to me.

I was born in the flames of a city on fire: London in the Blitz. When I was four, my mother left and never came back. My adoptive parents changed my name, altered my history, and told me I came from a children's home in London and my birth parents had been killed in the war. As unhappy as I was with these people, I thought that misery went with the territory of being adopted, with never knowing your own family. That was before I found out accidentally at the age of twenty-five that my adoptive mother was the sister of my birth mother and that my favorite "aunt" was actually my birth mother. While I looked after demented elderly women, I also began to experience a series of flashbacks that revealed my adoptive father had sexually molested me until I was eight years old. These revelations made me feel at home in what often feels to me like a whole nation of unmothered children.

These insights also give sense to my Alzheimer's work. Being surrounded by people with fractured memories and histories holds no fears for me. Sitting with the elderly as they weep for mothering and cry with the fear of abandonment does not threaten me. In fact, I feel strongly that, as I help them on their journey to comfort and healing before their deaths, I have helped that wounded part of myself. Sometimes people ask me how I can do this work—as if I were understudy to Mother Teresa. To them I have to answer, "How could I not? Alzheimer's has blessed me."

Having lived among other cultures, I find that Alzheimer's seems like one more culture to learn. I soon discovered that little help was available from the world of medicine. I had to learn the culture by living among people with Alzheimer's. I listened, I "hung out," I watched, I practiced my communication skills, and I began to understand something of what people with Alzheimer's want us to know.

I'm sure there is more to learn; I'm sure I have not been the best pupil. But what I know is what those with Alzheimer's have taught me, and what I don't know are those things I did not pay enough attention to. This book represents what I've learned so far. To my many teachers in my life of blessings, thank you.

—————————— Chapter 1 ——————————

Light for
the Journey

If you suspect or have recently discovered that someone you care about has Alzheimer's disease, you are about to undergo a profound journey. Alzheimer's disease affects not only the person who has it but also everyone who is concerned about that person. The disease becomes a rite of passage for all involved.

My hope is that this book will help you through this journey by providing the knowledge, guidance, and tools you will need. It does not have all the answers, since Alzheimer's disease and family journeys are intensely unique passages, but it may bring light to an area of darkness.

You will find in the following pages not only the practical hands-on help you need, but also an honest examination of how we may usefully deal with the crisis of love and the central problems that Alzheimer's brings about. Using many lessons gathered from the self-help movement, you will also learn how to avoid those traps that have destroyed many Alzheimer caregivers.

The Crisis of Love

The process of Alzheimer's disease is connected with losses, difficulties, and agonies. The central difficulty, however, and one that has been largely ignored by Alzheimer professionals, is the crisis of dysfunctional caregiving. It is not that Alzheimer's disease itself is so unrelentingly consuming; what are so destructive are the difficult emotional issues that Alzheimer's raises and that many people do not address.

Many of the stories you may have heard surrounding Alzheimer's disease are dark projections of people lost in the dysfunctional patterns that Alzheimer's brings to family relationships. All too often, such caregivers fail to listen to or observe their family member with Alzheimer's, and thus they never learn what is really needed.

The dysfunctional aspect of caregiving has been allowed to become the so-called norm of Alzheimer care. As a society, we have begun to recognize such dysfunction in other relationships, but we have avoided looking at it in Alzheimer's caregiving. Alzheimer's disease touches us at the very root of our deepest, darkest terrors. Most people have a fear of being helpless, of becoming totally dependent on others, of losing control, of being demeaned by a disease that may cause loss of mind or of control of basic bodily functions. Our societal dread of this illness means we have been willing to accept dysfunctional caregiving, simply because most people want to avoid looking at Alzheimer's at all.

We can no longer ignore this aspect of Alzheimer's. Too many caregivers are dying, and too many people with Alzheimer's are suffering at the hands of their caregivers. It is time to change that, and you can change it for yourself. You can change it by becoming a good caregiver to yourself, by being kind to yourself.

Alzheimer's disease brings us all face to face with the central crisis in our society: the crisis in which the parent does not meet the love needs of the child. We live in a society of the emotionally orphaned. However, even if you have been one of those millions of orphans who never experienced enough love, you can still learn to become a good caregiver and, in doing so, *you will become healed*. This is the most powerful message that Alzheimer's disease carries in the heart of its own darkness: the disease itself can become a source of light and love.

Remember, however, the warning of Trappist monk Thomas Merton: "He who attempts to act and do things for others. . .

without deepening his own self understanding, freedom, integrity and capacity to love, will not have anything to give others."

This book is not only about the nuts-and-bolts of Alzheimer's caregiving—although there are enough of those in these pages to build a battleship. It is about the ways in which you may deepen your own self-understanding, freedom, integrity, and capacity to love. It is about awakening to this journey as it becomes a spiritual pathway.

This book distills the experiences of hundreds of caregivers facing a wide range of Alzheimer issues. It deals with the all-too-familiar losses of the disease and reveals what remains hopeful, rewarding, and possible.

There are a few things you probably do not know about Alzheimer's disease:

- Most people do not lose their memories as much as they lose *reliable access* to their memories—an important difference.
- Many people with Alzheimer's never want to run away from home and never get lost or go wandering.
- Many people with Alzheimer's never experience those fits of rage often attributed to the disease; if they do, this is a short-lived phase. Nearly all anger in Alzheimer's is reactive, not irrational: it has causes that can be addressed.
- Most people need never become incontinent.
- Very few people with Alzheimer's die helplessly curled up in bed. Most die of the usual diseases of old age after remaining reasonably active until the end.
- The sense of humor survives, and the pleasures of life remain appreciated by many.
- Love always makes a difference, even if the person with Alzheimer's does not remember your name.

The most important thing, and one hardly anyone acknowledges, is that emotional growth is still possible for people with Alzheimer's. They are still capable of working on their life issues and resolving them. Attaining peace is, after all, the goal of most human beings, sick or well, demented or not, and such resolution remains entirely possible for the person with Alzheimer's.

Ignorance, bigotry, and cowardice surround this illness, even in the medical profession. Because Alzheimer's disease cannot be treated or cured right now, the most we can offer is to relate meaningfully to the person who has dementia.

The medical model of care does not include the art of relationship with the Alzheimer's patient; it concentrates largely on containment, control, feeding, and grooming. Being task-centered instead of person-centered, modern medicine too often ignores the essential personhood of the one who has Alzheimer's disease.

Family life, however, requires interpersonal dealings, and this book will teach you the art of relationship with the person you are caring for. You will undoubtedly face losses and hard times during the process, and this book cannot save you from them. It can, however, save you from drowning in them and show you how to use this struggle to find meaning and purpose in the journey.

The Journey of Caregiving

How you choose to approach this journey is highly personal. No one can make you do it well, just as no one can make you learn the language and customs of a foreign country. However, just as learning the language makes foreign travel much more rewarding and meaningful, "learning Alzheimer's disease" can make this difficult rite of passage a meaningful and even a fulfilling experience.

Alzheimer's changes people profoundly, and these changes are usually painful to observe. But an important thing to understand is that you will not lose your relationship with the person you are caring for, although you may have to allow your role in this relationship to change. This kind of change can bring about entirely new relationship dynamics, which are achieved only through a willingness to face pain and travel through it.

There is no "why?" that can be answered. Alzheimer's disease is not punishment, nor is it deserved by anyone or brought about by bad behavior or sins of omission. It is not sent as divine retribution. Diseases simply happen. They exist in the world and people get them for the complex and mysterious reasons that control such events. The most useful question you can ask yourself is not "why?" but "how?" "How am I to undertake this journey?" "How shall I learn what to do?" "How shall I cope?" These are useful questions. If your life is one of avoidance, blame, and denial about important issues, this passage will be unbearably painful, but if you face it through, you can find great joy even within the pain.

You may be fearful because you have never been good at dealing with crisis. You may be worried because you have never much liked the person you must care for and cannot imagine becoming a loving caregiver. Or, you may feel that because you liked this person so much before, you cannot bear to witness the prospective changes.

Either way, you *can* learn to become a good caregiver. You can use this hard and sometimes dark journey as a tool for your own transformation. All struggles provide an opportunity for change. In fact, the Chinese written language uses a character for "crisis" that also means "opportunity."

There will be times of sorrow. After all, a diagnosis of Alzheimer's disease will seem as though death has sent its calling card. You may feel overwhelmed by the situation at first, but that will pass.

Alzheimer's disease will take you through periods of darkness, but it can also include times of joy and laughter, love and fun. Alzheimer's demands change, and if you resist that change, you will suffer the consequences. Most of the suffering associated with Alzheimer's disease is among caregivers who refuse to change and meet the conditions of the disease. Those who try to hold on to the past are most likely to feel irretrievably angry or guilty. The willingness to change will offer you peace and resolution, and it will bring about profound differences in your relationship with the impaired person, in other family members, and, most of all, in yourself.

One of the most important gifts you can give yourself is to be patient with yourself from the beginning. Being hard on yourself uses up your energy and weighs down your heart. There is no perfect way to be an Alzheimer's caregiver. There is only a continuing learning process in the context of who you are. Even when you get it wrong, you will not do much harm. People with Alzheimer's do not break easily. And, best of all, the very nature of their disease means they forget your mistakes. Every day is a new beginning; take that as a blessing.

An Opportunity for Self-Discovery

New knowledge, new ways to relate, and new skills will bring you strength and self-discovery. Through this experience, you will be faced with family issues, sibling rivalries, and other struggles, and you will learn ways to deal with them.

Through caregiving, you will learn the secrets of decoding Alzheimer language and behavior and discover how to use them in a constructive way. The problem behaviors associated with the disease are often simply the ways in which the person with Alzheimer's is trying to communicate his or her needs to others. As you become a skillful caregiver, you will learn the secrets of defusing problems and be able to relate in a new and powerful way to the sick person. You will discover how to deal with the common problems of caregiving, how to find help, and, if you should come to it, how to make wise decisions about placement into institutional care. You will learn to change with changing situations, to forgive yourself, and to find meaning and happiness in the here and now.

Like any other task, becoming an Alzheimer caregiver requires you to learn special skills. This book will teach you much of what you need to know and lead you toward the changes you may have to undergo. Amazingly enough, if you are willing to make those changes and learn those skills, you will find that this will become a powerful spiritual and psychological pathway for you. You will find strengths you did not imagine you had, and they will be there for you to draw on the rest of your life.

Coping Mechanisms

Nothing, of course, removes all the darkness of the journey. No one could ever say that Alzheimer's is a good disease, and that is not the message of this book. The message is that the destructive gloom-and-doom approach gets us nowhere and gives us nothing.

Negativity and despair usually cover up the fact that a caregiver is refusing to change and is actually addicted to the stress of caregiving. You do not need to fall prey to that trap. Use this book as you would use a dictionary and guidebook when you visit a foreign country. No place is quite as foreign as Alzheimer's, and yet, even there, we can find guides and interpreters who can at least help us understand. Knowledge will be your light, and other sources of light will come from a sense of humor, love from your friends, support from other caregivers, and from the simple effort not to take all this so seriously.

Laugh whenever you can, hug as much as you can, and remember that love is the only useful management tool.

Do not let Alzheimer's become a morass into which you fall. Plenty of people will be willing to push you into it. After all, if you are coping, people who cannot cope or are afraid even to talk about the illness or be around it feel even worse about themselves. Avoid the doomsayers and gloom-carriers; their stock-in-trade is I-told-you-so helplessness. If your old friends cannot support your journey in a positive way, get new ones who can. Love yourself and treat yourself kindly.

While you are learning how to change, how to serve, and how to help, give yourself as much devotion as you give the person you look after. Keep a journal in which you are as truthful as you can be. As well as being a useful outlet for unmentionable feelings, a journal will gradually accumulate your knowledge and help you see how your journey progresses. Remember, whenever you feel overwhelmed, it is not Alzheimer's that overwhelms you; it is just today, and today will pass. You do not have to wait until the rite of passage is over before you can relax and have fun.

Most of all, you are the only expert. No one else knows this person you care for as you do. No one can tell what the best care is or why something is happening as well as you. Trust your own judgment.

Pay close attention to your spiritual life and allow it to help you through this rite of passage. Spiritual life does not refer to any particular religion or discipline but to a profound sense of being that supports you at the deepest level, including your sense of connection with the world around you. If you do all you can to feed the spiritual—through pursuing serenity, meditation, prayer, the peace of nature, therapy—you can avoid falling into constant crisis.

Even though the disease itself cannot yet be healed, you have the ability to make choices that lead you out of despair. You can heal your own relationship with this person, if need be, and heal your own lack of love in former times. These are the ordinary miracles of learning to be a caregiver.

As a caregiver, you can cope well or badly. You have that choice. Even doing badly on individual days does not mean you are stuck with coping badly.

It doesn't even matter if you feel that circumstances are forcing you into caregiving. No matter how reluctant you feel, you can learn to do this well.

Caring for someone with Alzheimer's disease is difficult, but you need to know that you can learn to do it and find deep, meaningful satisfaction in doing it well. You can grow spiritually and become a much more profound person who is no longer afraid of the journey ahead.

Nothing we learn as caregivers is wasted. It all enters the heart and mind to be stored and used throughout our lives. Even the fears we have at the beginning bring us new knowledge. After learning to become a good caregiver, you will no longer fear Alzheimer's itself. Don't let anyone tell you that you can't do this. Most people have no idea how to cope with dementia. Even doctors and nurses don't know how, and they're often the first to discourage you.

This is a profound journey into the heart of unconditional love. It is a journey on the outer edges of human experience, into largely unmapped territory. You will learn things you never imagined.

If you decide to become a member of that rare and honorable band, those who cope with dementia, congratulations. Our society may not understand, may stand back from you in pity, but you are part of a great army of quiet workers for light and love in this world. There are many of us. We will find each other, and we will help each other. Together we are joining in the task to bring some light to dealing with Alzheimer's disease, instead of cursing the darkness.

Chapter 2

The Caring Bystander

The years before a definite diagnosis of Alzheimer's are often frustrating and exhausting for family members who may suspect that something is wrong without being able to put their finger on it. Family members will often jump to the conclusion that their loved one has Alzheimer's disease. As this chapter will show, however, it is impossible to know from observation whether a person actually has Alzheimer's or if their problems have some other cause.

Long before a person is diagnosed as having Alzheimer's disease, there are usually small indicators. These signs often puzzle or alarm family members, but until they have accumulated sufficiently to cause major disquiet, their significance is not really understood. It is only in retrospect that these signposts can be seen as foreshadowing Alzheimer's, and perhaps they were not actually signposts at all. We are inclined to attribute personal peculiarities to the presence of disease when they might simply be individual idiosyncrasies.

Q: We think Mother has Alzheimer's disease. Ever since my father died, she has become more and more forgetful. She used to be very sociable and always played bridge with her friends at least two afternoons a week. Now she says she doesn't feel like seeing her friends anymore. Does she have Alzheimer's disease?

A: There is no simple answer to such a question. From the facts presented, your mother could be suffering from anything from grief to Alzheimer's disease. Grief can cause memory problems just as Alzheimer's can.

It is important not to jump to the conclusion that she has Alzheimer's, for a variety of reasons. The most important, of course, is that she may well not have it. In Western societies such a conclusion often leads families to give up on their elders, assuming that they have an untreatable illness.

Your mother does need your help. She may be trapped in depression and unable to transcend grief at the loss of her life partner. All the things you describe—withdrawing, memory problems, a drop in her personal standards for herself—could be caused by grief. Equally, she may have some other illness, treatable and curable. Or, you may find that, just as you fear, she does have Alzheimer's.

Try to get her to see her doctor. Perhaps you can accompany her and discuss your observations together so that her doctor can judge what the next steps should be. A physical exam is the most sensible place to start.

If she refuses, accept that you cannot force her. Be prepared to stand by to offer as much help as she needs. Show your concern as kindly as possible. Try to talk with her friends and find out whether they will help support your mother with friendship.

Q: What should we look for if we think someone we know might have Alzheimer's?

A: Since dementia takes many forms, it is hard to list all the questionable behaviors that indicate its presence. And, even if they could be concretely defined, we could not be absolutely sure what they signified.

Most Alzheimer indicators are behaviors that accumulate until they interfere with normal life. Until that happens, we cannot in fact claim these behaviors as indicators of Alzheimer's. So-called Alzheimer symptoms can be signs of many other conditions. They can even be caused by medications. The average elderly person takes six medications for other medical conditions. Therefore, be alert to possible warning signs, but do not make any assumptions.

Following is a list of signs that indicate some problem exists, but not necessarily Alzheimer's. Typical problems that should alert us that a person needs some kind of help are:

- repeated car accidents
- getting lost
- seeming confused
- decreased ability to maintain usual lifestyle
- becoming unkempt
- no longer doing household tasks
- becoming unable to follow rational discussions
- unable to do paperwork
- dropping former interests for no apparent reason
- not recalling the previous day
- losing things

The real sign of trouble is when a number of the items on the above list accumulate.

Q: How can you tell for sure that someone has Alzheimer's?

A: Not easily. The final diagnosis of Alzheimer's disease is made only after all other possibilities have been eliminated. It is a diagnosis that basically says, "We can't find anything else that fits, so we can now assume this must be Alzheimer's disease."

The diagnosis is usually stated to be "a dementia of the Alzheimer type," sometimes shortened to DAT. If someone you know exhibits a number of the signs discussed, proper medical investigation is needed. These signs are warnings that something is wrong, whether that something is Alzheimer's or depression or liver disease.

Every individual with Alzheimer's has a personal style of presenting the disease. These many variations are what cause confusion and questions among family members. Given that Alzheimer sufferers have certain universal problems—the most obvious being memory loss—they also vary widely, so much so that some medical experts suggest there may be several kinds of Alzheimer's disease. Some think this is not so much a specific disease as a collection of identifying behaviors and variable symptoms—in other words, a syndrome.

Q: We think my aunt has Alzheimer's. What should we do?

A: Encourage your aunt to get a complete checkup, including neurological testing, CT scans, and laboratory tests.

First, speak privately to her doctor so that your concerns are known, and so that the doctor may be alert to her attempts to cover up her problems.

This will enable her doctor to run a dementia test while interviewing her. If she's not ready for that, be prepared to stand by and help her until she is ready.

Q: I want my husband to be tested for Alzheimer's, but he says there's nothing wrong with him. How can I make him get tested?

A: It is typical for Alzheimer patients to deny there is anything wrong with them, often in a confident and convincing manner. Many family members report their frustration over this.

"I told the doctor my husband was having severe memory problems, but he just asked him if he ever forgot anything and my husband said cheerfully, 'Oh no, in fact I've got a great memory.' Frankly, I could have killed the pair of them!" reports one frustrated wife.

It was a year later before her husband was finally diagnosed, and this was only after she insisted on a full Alzheimer workup from a neurologist. Some families have communication problems with their doctors over their early suspicions, sometimes being dismissed with vague phrases like, "What can you expect at his age?" or "There may be a little senility there."

There are many good doctors and it is essential to have one when dealing with Alzheimer's, even if this means changing physicians. Since Alzheimer's is so variable, you need an experienced doctor to deal with it, one who respects elders and believes they deserve the best medical treatment appropriate for their well-being.

Make an appointment yourself with your husband's doctor. Take with you a written account of what you've observed. This will be one way of starting what may well be a long road toward diagnosis.

Meanwhile, be patient, and understand that fear makes your husband deny he has problems. The more understanding you are, the safer he will feel. Then he may be able to allow himself to undergo the diagnostic process.

It is not too early for you to join an Alzheimer's support group. That way, you will get the support you need from others who know your situation well from their own experience. They will help you to go through the process ahead.

Q: *Our grandmother has some memory problems, but it doesn't seem too bad yet. Does this mean she has Alzheimer's? At what point does a little forgetfulness turn into Alzheimer's? How long should we wait?*

A: Your grandmother's memory problems may be just that—simple lapses of memory. Possibly with your help and support, she may continue to live her life without becoming too disabled by memory lapses.

As we have already observed, memory problems alone do not signify the presence of Alzheimer's. While it is true that Alzheimer's always comes with memory problems, as well as other problems, a little forgetfulness does not signify the presence of disease. It has become politically incorrect these days to admit that increasing age is often accompanied by increasing memory problems, but my observations of elders in the past ten years indicate that there is a certain truth in this.

The truth, however, is more complex than simply saying that age leads to memory problems. Research shows that elders who study may do as well as their younger classmates. Their processing of memory is different, but not less efficient for learning purposes. Most elders have long given up scholastic-type studies, however, and are therefore out of practice with learning.

The lifestyle of elders also tends to produce less reliance on memory function. When the routine of work is left behind, there are fewer indicators to remind people of the differences in days and often less stimulation from the outside world.

There is also the vexed question of medications. The tragedy and disgrace of modern medication practice is that many medications cause memory problems, chief among them the medications for the most common medical conditions affecting elders—heart, blood pressure, glaucoma, and diabetes medications being the worst.

Thus, many factors combine in later life to create a situation where memory awareness is not supported. This may be what is happening to your grandmother. There is also another factor: some elders are absorbed in their inner life, carrying out a complex life review that does not allow much focus on the present and outer life. Keep a watchful eye on your grandmother, because only time will tell. Don't assume she is developing Alzheimer's. That may not be true. Help her live stress-free.

Q: Do people who are getting Alzheimer's know there's something wrong?

A: After working with many Alzheimer sufferers and talking with their families, it is obvious to me that there is a much earlier phase than the one normally identified as "early stage." This is the "invisible phase." It covers the period of time in which only the individual concerned knows or suspects that there is something wrong within. This phase may last many years.

One woman, diagnosed at seventy-four, had written in her diaries twenty years earlier that she was experiencing problems with her thinking. She described "these terrible absentmindednesses" that involved both problems of memory and problems in thinking things through.

Another woman, a Jungian psychologist, noted a series of dreams she had thirty years before being diagnosed with Alzheimer's. In these dreams doctors told her she had an incurable brain disease. She did not interpret these dreams literally at the time, and it was only her later illness which retrospectively suggests that she should have.

There is much anecdotal evidence like these examples that suggest interesting questions about how some people have deep inner knowledge of their true state of health, even before any signs of illness are visible to others. The invisible phase, during which the individual lives with the growing awareness that something is wrong, gradually becomes evident in behavior changes.

Often, these changes are inexplicable at the time. An outgoing, gregarious man gave up his social life entirely, telling his wife he "just could not be bothered." At the time, she put it down to the demands of his work, but later she saw it as the beginning of Alzheimer's disease. Another woman stopped playing mah-jongg with her friends. When her son asked her why, she answered vaguely, "Oh, I don't like those people anymore."

Some people show no outward signs that they are troubled, and yet later discoveries reveal that they were aware of their encroaching illness. One woman started in her early forties to collect articles on memory loss, even though she worked at a demanding job until retirement and was not actually diagnosed until she was eighty. Her family discovered her secret cache of clippings after she went into skilled nursing care.

Other signs are much more outward. A man who never drank to excess began to drink heavily and to throw temper tantrums at home. This period extended for several years, during which his wife was frantic. "I thought my Bill hated me. I thought he was going to leave me. He used to scream at me and throw his dinner plate against the wall. I had no idea what was going on at that time." Only when Bill was finally diagnosed with Alzheimer's disease did his wife understand he had been reacting in sheer terror to his knowledge that he was losing control within. Either because of denial or a sense of terror that he could not reveal, or simply because he did not know the nature of what was going on, he never spoke about it to his wife. When he was finally diagnosed and the doctor broke the news to him and his wife together, Bill said, "Thank God! Oh, thank God! I thought I was going crazy!"

This is not an uncommon reaction among Alzheimer sufferers. While their families are afraid to mention the word "Alzheimer's" to them, they themselves are often convinced they are going mad or becoming stupid and they cannot talk about their unformulated fears and feelings. Instead, they act them out.

Many behavior changes may mark the invisible phase, some of which have already been mentioned:

- development of intense suspicion and fear of others
- inability to follow through on projects, such as tending a garden, sewing something, or organizing an event
- problems following thoughts through
- the onset of depression
- sudden onset of drinking bouts in a person not previously given to drinking
- inability to continue to handle responsibilities in work, community, or family affairs
- having gaps of logic that cannot be filled no matter how often others explain them
- outbreaks of irrational rage
- responding with hostility for no apparent reason
- unbelievable stories of bad things done by others
- throwing scenes in public places, like banks or stores; such outbursts are actually due to inability to process information

All these signs could indicate problems with thought processes and the gradual failure of rational thinking ability, together with emotional attrition.

Q: We always used to think old people got forgetful. Now they always say it's Alzheimer's. Is it really a disease?

A: Many elderly people routinely have some problems with memory that do not become a major pathological feature of their lives. It is also common for the elderly who are entering their dying process—which may take several years in the case of someone in their eighties or nineties—to be forgetful. This is much more benign than the global forgetting and memory failures of Alzheimer's.

We forget, or do not understand, how much the elderly are involved in inner work of resolution and reconciliation. We assume that the shape of life for the elderly ought to be the same as it has always been and that anything different can only be a sign of a declining lifestyle.

This is certainly better than assuming that all old people should retire to nursing homes. These days, thankfully, people may age in any style they choose and remain as active and youthful as they feel capable of being. Being over sixty does not mean the end of sexual activity, sports, study, or personal growth.

People are free to be who they are. However, since we know so little about aging—and are deeply reluctant to learn—we know almost nothing about its psychological and spiritual processes.

I have been told by many elders—both those with dementia and those in good health—that they experience an intensification of memory. Moments flash into their consciousness, bringing back a time, a moment, an event of many years before in absolute clarity—the smell, the color, the clothing and words of people they had not thought of for many decades.

This kind of memory process occurs as we age. I believe it starts in the fifties, intensifying year by year. I have seen no reference to this in any literature, but I have observed it myself and my observations have been confirmed by a number of elders.

This is part of the process of reviewing and reconciling life, and those with dementia also experience this form of memory flashback. People with dementia may be unaware that it is memory; the flashback is experienced as actually happening in the moment.

It becomes steadily more evident that memory is not a simple matter of filed references, either recalled or forgotten. Instead, memory is an organic process with purpose and meaning. Even among those who are technically regarded as suffering from memory loss, memory is a vivid and meaningful part of life.

Remember, people with dementia do not suffer from memory loss. They suffer *unreliable memory access.*

Q: My mother has started avoiding people, even family members. Last month her sister came to visit and my mother refused even to come out of her room the whole time her sister was here. It's really embarrassing and I don't understand it at all. What is wrong with her?

A: Often, the only sign of coming trouble with Alzheimer's disease is a mood change—depression or anxiety or increasing dependence even over very small things.

However, these could also be signs of depression as an illness in itself, or a response to other factors in the environment. Not knowing exactly what these changes mean leads to greater emotional stress both for family members and for the person who may be manifesting the first visible signs of disease.

One woman of seventy-four was told by her youngest son to become more independent at a time when, unknown to him, she was reminding herself who her own children were by writing memos. "My youngest son is Myron and he teaches high school. My oldest son is Deiter and he's a doctor in Chicago." Her sudden increased dependency came out of her knowledge that she was losing her memory.

Another family identified their mother's early dementia as

"Mother's nerves" and explained her tears and tantrums as a sign that she and their father were not enjoying their retirement. As true as that observation was, it was far from being the real story of what was happening. They tried to deal with their mother's growing incapacity by bringing in household help, but their mother would fire the help behind their backs. She was not ready to reveal her neediness other than to family members, who in turn were not ready to acknowledge it.

The best thing you can do for your mother right now is to stand by her and assure her of your support. This helps her to feel that, if necessary, she can trust you and rely on you. Keep a close watch on her and write down what you see. These notes will help her doctor understand what is happening to her.

Q: How long does it take for someone to enter the first or early stage of Alzheimer's?

A: Although the common medical term for the cumulative gathering of visible symptoms is *early stage Alzheimer's*, this is not necessarily a correct description. Family members must not think it literally means the disease is in its beginnings.

Experts do not know when Alzheimer's really begins. Perhaps a person is born with the disease already present, or perhaps it is triggered at some point through causes not yet established.

After the invisible stage comes the *visible early stage*. During this time, which again may extend for many years or a few months, the family sees a number of disquieting signs accumulating. These are likely to include some or all of the following:
- overall inability to function as well as before
- deterioration in personal appearance
- decline in personal hygiene
- wearing odd combinations of clothing
- incapacity to deal with household bills and documents
- dropping old friendships and social patterns
- avoiding contact even with close family members

- becoming increasingly dependent
- staying in bed for long periods for no apparent reason
- becoming fearful or anxious for no apparent reason
- telling unlikely stories about strange events
- calling the police for no valid reason
- having domestic accidents, such as leaving pots burning on the stove or leaving appliances on
- marked change in sleep patterns
- getting lost while driving or having a series of unaccounted-for car accidents
- being unable to account for the day's activities
- showing inconsistencies of memory or behavior
- lack of food in the refrigerator or cupboards
- inability to shop
- hoarding one kind of food, such as eighteen tins of beans or eight boxes of cookies
- mood changes seemingly unrelated to external events

This list could be endless, since any kind of variation might appear in any individual. Basically, these signs add up to decreasing competency in daily life, increasing memory problems that affect basic functioning, and signs of emotional distress. They continue the list of global losses we noted as the first signs of trouble.

Obviously, there are many possible reasons for these developments, which is why it is important to persuade the person to seek help.

Q: We think our dad might be getting Alzheimer's. Whenever we try to help him, he says he's doing fine and doesn't need us. He's a very independent man and of course we want to respect that, but we need to know when to intervene.

A: This can be the hardest thing of all, since most families try to respect the desire of members to remain independent as long as possible. Like you, they do not want to interfere. However, in general, you need to know that families usually intervene too late rather than too soon. It is almost unknown for a family to intervene inappropriately early.

You can be sure that by the time you have noticed signs of distress accumulating, you are dealing with an important problem. Even when the whole family recognizes there is a problem, they often hesitate to interfere until the disease becomes much more advanced.

If this is your case, it would be a good idea for all family members to talk about how you can ensure life quality, tactful help, and discreet monitoring of your father. Consider a shopping plan, a visiting plan, a meal schedule, help with household papers and bills, and so on.

It is not a kindness to leave him to cope beyond his capacity to do so. It places a heavy burden on him and undoubtedly adds to his stress tremendously. Demented people cannot run their own lives. It is that simple.

The hard part is to know exactly how to intervene. It's natural for your father to resent your butting in. Whatever their degree of stress, people never thank you for this. They never say, "You're right. I can't run my own life. I'm so grateful you want to take it over for me!"

Get family members together to discuss what you are seeing. Everyone should have input into this discussion. This is useful as a reality check for the whole family. This is important since the early visible stages are often somewhat nebulous—a fading of capacity rather than a clearly delineated set of circumstances.

If some members of your family are in doubt about what they are seeing, it is sometimes helpful for everyone to make a list of the problems. Note each incident or symptom and discuss whether they add up to illness. Normal idiosyncrasies should be left off the list. You are looking for changes that indicate decline, a growing inability to manage life as before. When only one or two indicators are found, assume that this slight decline is within a range of normal aging changes, and stop worrying. If the list is long, obviously this indicates problems.

Q: My grandmother got pretty forgetful before she died, and this was before people were talking about Alzheimer's. She was pretty healthy until the last two years of her life. She died at eighty-nine. Could she have had Alzheimer's?

A: In our new awareness of Alzheimer's, it is important not to label all such withdrawals as dementia. A woman of ninety begins forgetting names and addresses because she is inwardly concentrating on setting her primary relationships to peace.

This process does not deserve the label of Alzheimer's disease. There really are days when it doesn't matter who the president is or what the date is.

People's ignorance of the aging and dying process leads them to label all changes as pathological. After ten years of close contact with the very old, both healthy and infirm, it is clear to me that a great deal of inward work and concentration goes into this final process.

While this process is under way, it is normal for facts, time, and previous patterns of daily life to become irrelevant. This is not disease. It is the process of closure and often a time of great blessing. It asks of us our understanding and our acceptance.

Q: If someone gets Alzheimer's, should they be put into a nursing home?

A: Alzheimer's is not necessarily a reason to rush the ailing person into medical or nursing care. Increasing family support could help to keep the person coping with limited independence. Family members could take over certain household tasks or duties and see whether the situation gets better or worse or holds steady at a plateau.

Unless an actual trauma of some kind occurs, family members need not hurry into life-changing decisions. When trauma does occur, however, often a rapid decline results. At this point, full-time care may be necessary. Such care could be provided at home or in a small care home. Nursing home care is not required. In fact, nursing homes are often inappropriate for good dementia

care. Families should look at all the possibilities, rather than immediately assuming that a nursing home is the answer.

The contents of this chapter illustrate how complicated family
life becomes when we suspect, but cannot be sure, that a loved
one may have Alzheimer's. The best course, when we are uncertain,
is to act like a caring friend, even if the person involved is one's
parent or spouse. The closer we are, the more we feel we have to
take charge. But until we know exactly what we are in charge of,
we are forced to remain in suspension.

This is especially hard for most people. We do not stand and
wait with great patience. Most of us would rather be doing than
being. This is one reason whey there are so many spiritual disci-
plines built around learning to be, rather than learning to do.

As the Vietnamese Buddhist monk Thich Nhat Hanh says,
"Don't just do something, sit there!" Being willing to sit there in
the right way is important. It means not trying to force the person
you care about to admit, confess, or agree there is something
wrong. It means intervening when necessary in a tactful, supportive way, using graciousness, not bullying. It means being
actively kind in order to create a sense of trust that might allow
that person finally to share the secret of Alzheimer's with you.

Most people have a difficult time admitting that there is something seriously wrong with their lives. People are often very careful
about whom they reveal their health secrets to, such as having
cancer or being HIV-positive.

This is even more true for our elders, most of whom were
brought up to believe that you never tell others your secret issues
and never discuss things like your terminal illnesses. Add to this
habit of secrecy the immense extra shadow we cast around mental
health issues, and you can see why it might take a long time for
someone you care about to be able to broach the subject with you.

Your loving and tactful attitude will create a blanket of safety
that might encourage such risk-taking. Even if this is your own
mother or your own father, try to be a supportive friend throughout
the years by standing by.

Chapter 3

Alzheimer's Up to Date

The first thing to know about Alzheimer's is that almost nothing is really known about it—not the causes, not the treatments, certainly not the cure. In fact, some respected researchers have recently raised the question of whether Alzheimer's disease is actually a disease at all or merely an extreme edge of the natural aging process.

Much of what you hear about Alzheimer's disease is repetition of not-yet-established "facts," medical myths that are often given spurious authority simply by dint of being repeated often. For those researchers who are really in the heart of the exploration of Alzheimer's, it is commonly accepted that very little is known and that the biggest problem is that we do not really know what normal old age looks like. This extreme lack of knowledge has led to a number of false trails in the search for the truth about Alzheimer's disease, and undoubtedly there is far to go.

Q: What is Alzheimer's disease?

A: The following is the Alzheimer's Association's official statement on Alzheimer's disease: "Alzheimer's disease is a progressive degenerative disease that attacks the brain and results in impaired memory, thinking, and behavior. It is considered to be one of the most common forms of dementia."

It is not really established fact that Alzheimer's is the most common form of dementia, but this is an often repeated statement. The American Psychiatric Association's definition of Alzheimer's disease, contained in the *Diagnostic and Statistical Manual*, fourth edition, extends that explanation a little more fully:

> The essential feature of the presence of Dementia of insidious onset and gradual progressive course for which all other specific causes have been excluded by the history, physical examination, and laboratory tests.

> The Dementia involves a multifaceted loss of intellectual abilities, such as memory, judgment, abstract thought, and other higher cortical functions, and changes in personality and behavior.

Q: Is Alzheimer's a form of insanity?

A: No. Alzheimer's is not a mental illness. It is a physical illness that causes a degeneration of the organic structure of the brain. This, in turn, impairs all the normal processes of the brain—memory, cognitive thinking, perception. It does not, however, cause insanity.

Therefore, it is not appropriate for people with dementia to be given psychotropic or antipsychotic medications. Neither is it appropriate to use the terminology of psychiatry to describe the actions and feelings of a person with dementia. To do so dehumanizes an intense personal ordeal. It deceives one into thinking there is no reason to try to understand what we see, hear, and feel from the person who is ill. People with Alzheimer's are working against all this to try to make sense of their daily lives.

Q: What's the difference between Alzheimer's disease and dementia?

A: Alzheimer's disease is one form of dementia, possibly the most common, or perhaps only the one most likely to be named as such.

There are a number of dementias of old age—some experts say fifty or more. The term *dementia* does not refer to a specific disease but to its symptoms. Just as the presence of jaundice indicates a disease of the liver, so dementia indicates a disease of thinking function, the reason for which has to be established.

Dementia is a syndrome of behaviors and symptoms that show distorted, dysfunctional, and damaged thinking processes, as well as other problems such as memory loss. There are many causes of dementia, both temporary and curable, long-term and incurable. Right now, Alzheimer's disease is probably the best known, although it is likely that many of the people said to have Alzheimer's disease may not in fact have it.

Q: Can you get Alzheimer's through stress? A friend said she read that somewhere.

A: Medical science does not address the role of stress in the development of Alzheimer's. However, from ten years of personal observation of elders with Alzheimer's and interaction with their families, I would say that experientially a link between Alzheimer's and stress exists. While I would not go so far as to say that stress actually causes Alzheimer's, I would say that it can hasten its onset and definitely increases its severity. Undoubtedly, the link between the two is complex.

Elders often suffer severe losses in old age for which they get very little support: loss of life partners, loss of home through relocation or illness, loss of friends, loss of personal abilities. Often there is nowhere for them to turn and no way they can fill the gaps without skilled help from others.

That help is often unavailable. There are few peer group programs for elders to support each other and little funding in mental health programs for elders. Through these accumulating traumas, any tendency toward illnesses like Alzheimer's is made increasingly more likely to become reality.

May there be a stronger link between Alzheimer's and stress than research has fully established? This question remains largely unexplored. We do know that stress causes memory problems by actually destroying memory cells. This stress is of a temporary nature, and its effects are reparable. If stress remains constant and unrelenting, we simply do not know whether it can lead to permanent memory problems. I can say from my own observations that Alzheimer's patients have experienced an unusually high degree of stress in their lives, often from birth onward.

In a fifty-four-bed Alzheimer unit in Alameda, California, I observed that a significantly high number of the residents had been orphaned young, abandoned, brought up in abusive circumstances, and lived dramatically difficult lives. This suggests that further examination of these factors needs to be carried out.

Removing stress is probably not the answer to preventing the disease, not to mention how difficult it would be to eliminate all stress. But helping people to learn how to deal with stress might be one step.

Q: What happens in Alzheimer's?

A: Alzheimer's is usually described as having early, middle, and late stages (or first, second, and terminal). Some experts divide it up more minutely, into as many as nine stages depending on the degree of impairment observed.

The visible onset of the early stage of Alzheimer's disease is usually gradual and typically features a number of problems, the most noticeable involving the growing inability to access memory reliably. Usually there are also losses in ability to think cognitively—to think things through logically—and gradual loss of intellectual capacity. As these functions are increasingly affected, there is a growing inability to manage daily life efficiently. For example, job performance drops; the person gets lost while driving. Other signs may include mood changes, unwillingness to go out or inability to initiate anything. The person often is unable to assess the extent of these changes, or may blame others.

Since everyone manifests Alzheimer's in his or her own way,

the specific problems of the early stage vary. One woman lost the ability to read and write at the beginning of her illness, for example, while another seriously impaired woman could still read and write well into the course of her illness.

The middle or second stage shows increases in all problems so far presented. It is in this often extended stage that many of the so-called problem behaviors of Alzheimer's emerge: restlessness, changes in sleep patterns, agitation known as sundowning (because it comes on at the end of the day), wandering, rapid mood changes from weeping to anger, problems with perceptual-motor processes, impaired ability to communicate clearly, and a steadily increasing need for companionship and supervision around the clock.

This book will explore the tangible issues of these behaviors, which are due not so much to the presence of Alzheimer's as to the pressures the care environment places on the person's emotional and psychological needs.

The late or terminal stage, which typically lasts from one to three years, shows total loss of ability to run life. The person may become unable to recognize others, lose weight, and generally fail in overall functioning. Some people stop talking altogether. Some become bedridden and may become as care-dependent as infants.

By no means does everyone who gets Alzheimer's reach this stage. In fact, only about one in thirty people becomes so fully disabled. Perhaps it should be questioned whether this is truly the third stage or a particularly virulent and unusual form of disease impairment. The great majority of people who get Alzheimer's disease do not reach this third, or terminal, stage; they die of the normal diseases of age in the second stage.

Q: How long do people live once they develop Alzheimer's?

A: The course of the disease varies greatly. It can be anywhere from three to twenty-six years. The average survival rate from time of diagnosis is nine years.

31

The time of diagnosis, however, does not necessarily mark the beginning of the disease. As a general observation, in early-onset Alzheimer's—that is, Alzheimer's disease diagnosed in a significantly younger person—the course of the disease is often shorter and more severe.

It is unusual to develop Alzheimer's before sixty-five years of age, but it happens. The youngest person identified with Alzheimer's so far was twenty-seven. Early-onset Alzheimer's usually manifests in people in their thirties, forties, and fifties. It is usually associated with a particular genetic profile that is very unusual in Alzheimer's disease.

As a nonmedical bystander, I wonder why we do not designate these early-onset dementias as something other than Alzheimer's disease, rather than confuse the already difficult task of understanding the true Alzheimer's process.

Q: How many people have Alzheimer's disease?

A: Alzheimer's Association statistics claim that 10 percent of the population over sixty-five may have Alzheimer's, rising to 47 percent in people aged eighty-five and over. These figures must be regarded with some doubt, especially as the latter is based on one study alone. It is not enough to rest on such an extreme assertion, although it does make for good fund-raising appeal.

Furthermore, any figure that suggests that half of any given population, even one aged eighty-five years and older, is seriously ill must be regarded askance, unless we are to assume this is an extreme aspect of normal aging. This would demolish much of the case for differentiating Alzheimer's as a disease distinct from extreme aging—what we might call "toxic aging"—and would probably be a politically unacceptable stance to the Alzheimer's world at this point.

Q: What's the point of getting an official diagnosis when there's no treatment for Alzheimer's? Isn't that a needless expense?

A: For the majority of people over sixty-five who undertake the Alzheimer's workup, the cost is covered by Medicare. Apart from that, there are two excellent reasons for having the total Alzheimer's workup.

One is that this disease will not always be untreatable and incurable. Several major experimental drug programs are exploring the enhancement of brain process by using chemicals to replace missing or impaired brain chemistry. We are likely to see positive results from these programs soon.

The second reason is that there are a number of conditions that look like Alzheimer's disease but are not and can be cured. Fifteen to twenty percent of Alzheimer-like symptoms are actually caused by other curable or treatable medical conditions. Unfortunately, it is not unheard of for doctors to state on observation alone that an elder has Alzheimer's. The elder may in fact be struggling with another condition that could be treatable. For example, one woman whose doctor had said he considered her to have Alzheimer's disease later turned out to have water on the brain, which was then controlled by placement of a shunt in her skull. After this, many of her symptoms gradually disappeared. No diagnosis of Alzheimer's should be accepted merely on the opinion of one medical practitioner, unbacked by a total Alzheimer workup.

An additional reason, though sometimes unpopular with families, is that it is better to know as soon as possible what you are dealing with, even if it is Alzheimer's. The family can begin its education process rather than just stumbling through the next five years making life hard for themselves and the family member with dementia.

Q: *What would a full medical workup include?*

A: The full Alzheimer workup includes a complete physical, psychiatric, and neurological evaluation by experts in Alzheimer's disease. The physical includes a complete medical history, mental status test, and neuropsychological testing. It requires blood work, urinalysis, chest X ray, electroencephalography (EEG), computerized tomography (CT scan), and an electrocardiogram (EKG).

The staff involved are likely to include doctors, such as neurologists and psychiatrists, nurses and nursing aides experienced with dementia patients, and social workers. Since these specialists and staff are accustomed to dealing with people who are impaired by dementia, they are usually good at relating in a nonthreatening and comforting way to the person suspected of having Alzheimer's. Most of the procedures are not at all frightening or distressing. In fact, most people respond very well to the interest and concern being shown to them and may well enjoy the two or three days that this workup may take. The only part of the procedure that family members report as being distressing or frightening in some cases is the CT scan.

This battery of testing is done to exclude all other conditions that present dementia-like symptoms. Once all other identifiable conditions have been eliminated, a diagnosis will be given, usually two or three weeks later, after all the laboratory test results have been analyzed. The diagnosis is usually phrased as "a dementia of the Alzheimer type," or DAT, because it is impossible to diagnose Alzheimer's disease for sure.

It is often said that we can only establish the presence of Alzheimer's after death in an autopsy of the brain. The brain of a person who has died of Alzheimer's disease is reportedly identifiable by the presence of plaques and tangles that show physical degeneration of the brain. Recently, however, researchers have been faced with the problem that this evidence is not as easy to establish as was once thought.

Q: Okay, so the workup confirms a diagnosis of Alzheimer's. What now?

A: Currently, the diagnosis of Alzheimer's presents a situation in which there is neither treatment nor cure, but this could change literally at any moment with news of a breakthrough. Millions of dollars are being spent in the pursuit of its research and treatment.

Family members can do the following:
1. Educate themselves about how to make things easier for themselves and for the person with Alzheimer's instead of buying into the common societal fears about the disease.
2. Find out what local resources are available.
3. Get family members into local support groups and the person with Alzheimer's into contact with as many helpful resources as possible.

These steps are explored more fully in this book, but the main thing to keep in mind is not to give way to despair or fear. Other forms of help from natural medical resources are explained (see chapter 8), as well as personal growth processes that need to be undertaken by family members. People have a great deal of resistance to necessary growth, but undertaking it is the only way to make the Alzheimer's journey easier.

Q: Why are we hearing much more about Alzheimer's? Is there a rise in incidence? Is it different from senility?

A: The disease process has likely always been present in human populations. It was not named Alzheimer's until recently, but its appearance was similar enough for us to guess it was the same disease. Talk to any elderly person and you will hear about their grandmother or great-grandmother who became forgetful and had to be looked after.

Senility simply means "being demented because of age." The word *senile* actually comes from the Latin word for "sixty," so it means "sixtyish." Senility was merely an umbrella statement describing dementia without considering its cause or form.

One reason Alzheimer's seems so common is the publicity surrounding it. Most people have heard of it by now, and it is how most people would describe dementia. Another important factor is that more and more people are living longer, and the disease congregates in older populations. Therefore, statistically more people live with Alzheimer's disease today than in the past.

Whether a greater *percentage* of the population is living with Alzheimer's now is harder to establish. If we really do have a higher percentage of Alzheimer's now, we would have to ask what in particular could be causing such an increase. This seems to be a question that is not asked by the mainstream Alzheimer's world, probably because most research is being undertaken by those who are looking for drug solutions, with drug companies funding their research.

The big push in the mainstream Alzheimer's world is to find the magic bullet of medical cure, an approach that has notably failed in the realm of cancer research. This is why we must hope that a more flexible exploration of Alzheimer's, its causes and its treatment, becomes fashionable.

Why do we need such flexibility? Because the causes may be psychological, sociological, personal, and environmental, as much as medical. In my ten years of working closely with people with Alzheimer's, I have observed the following:

1. People with Alzheimer's have often had serious childhood problems.
2. Stress and trauma play major parts in the development of Alzheimer's.
3. Many Alzheimer sufferers fit a certain personality profile (see chapter 10).

Sociological factors may play a role as well, such as the fact that many elders live far from family and lack social support and help through the many severe crises and losses that pile up on elders— loss of partner, relocation, loss of personal abilities, and so on.

On the question of actual numbers, the Alzheimer's Association says 4 million Americans have Alzheimer's, and the number may rise to 20 million by the middle of the next century.

Q: Who gets Alzheimer's?

A: Just about anyone from anywhere—America, China, Europe, Samoa, India. So far, no society seems to be without its quota of people with Alzheimer's—except possibly those cultures in which the lifespan is very short, such as Chad or Laos.

No evidence establishes that intelligent and intellectual people are spared, nor are stupid and uneducated people spared. It is a democratic disease, cutting across all classes, occupations, and races.

Certain areas of the world show clusters of the disease: in Wales, in parts of Canada where aluminum deposits have polluted the water supply, and in the Marshall Islands, where an Alzheimer-like dementia afflicts many people, a dementia for which no cause has been established (although researchers are considering dietary factors and the fact that the Marshall Islands are downwind from the nuclear testing island of Bikini). In all these areas, Alzheimer's follows the same pattern of mainly afflicting people age sixty-five and older.

Q: How was Alzheimer's discovered?

A: Alzheimer's disease is named for Alois Alzheimer, a German physician working at a famous Swiss psychiatric institution, the Bergholzi Clinic, where he was a contemporary with Carl Jung. Alzheimer had a particular interest in pre-senile dementia, which he considered to have its cause in different factors from senile dementias, or those that develop after the age of sixty-five. In 1898 he wrote an exhaustive update on psychogeriatric disorders based on his research.

Alzheimer thought that pre-senile dementia had its origin in the physical degeneration of the brain itself, but that senile dementia came about through vascular problems. He regarded pre-senile and senile dementia as two entirely separate kinds of dementia.

Using a newly developed high-resolution microscope, Alzheimer carried out autopsies on patients who had been diagnosed with dementia during their life. He found evidence that is still considered to be the identifying factor in the autopsy confirmation of Alzheimer's disease—currently, the only definitive way of establishing that a person had Alzheimer's.

Alzheimer found deterioration of the physical system of the brain and considered this to be the sign of disease, but he did not realize that he had discovered a new disease and he did not name it himself. It was his medical director, Emil Kraeplin, who named the condition Alzheimer's disease in a textbook published in 1910.

Meanwhile, Alzheimer had written up his own research in a medical textbook, including what is regarded as the first documented case of Alzheimer's disease, that of a fifty-one-year-old woman who had been brought to see him by her husband. The woman suffered various impairments, as well as being unreasonably and unjustifiably jealous of her husband. She died within the year, and Alzheimer then conducted an autopsy of her brain. He found significant presence of tangles of fibers (neurofibrillary tangles) and clusters of degenerated nerve endings (neuritic plaques).

It was not until the late 1960s that researchers in the United States reexamined Alzheimer's work and began to diagnose certain specific forms of dementia as Alzheimer's disease.

There is an interesting subtext to the discovery of Alzheimer's disease. More recent researchers at the University of Florence in Italy have questioned whether Alzheimer's original case actually exhibited what is now regarded as Alzheimer's disease. The woman's autopsy results, they contend, had features that are atypical of the Alzheimer cases being recorded today. Another point is that Alzheimer himself would not recognize most of the cases we call Alzheimer's disease as being the same as those from which he drew his observations. He was looking at pre-senile dementia, which occurred specifically in younger people. The conclusions he drew were applied to those cases, since he regarded those older than sixty-five as having dementias caused by vascular problems.

Now, we typically regard Alzheimer's as a disease appearing in those over sixty-five years of age, and more especially in those over eighty. So, in a real way, the original disease identified by Alzheimer may not be the disease we now identify under his name.

Q: Why do we know so little about how to treat or cure Alzheimer's?

A: We know so little about Alzheimer's disease partly because we know little about the aging process, normal or abnormal. Few studies of the aging brain had been done prior to the current rise of Alzheimer's research. This means that the symptoms of Alzheimer's disease cannot be ruled out as symptoms of normal aging. This is one reason why we hear of possible causes that later evaporate as more research is done.

For example, are we right to label the forgetfulness of an ill woman in her mid-eighties as Alzheimer's disease? Maybe she is forgetful simply because of general debility. We really do not know the answer to such questions.

Since we cannot answer simple questions like these, it is even harder for us to know why people get Alzheimer's and how we can stop it. However, it is probably one of the most-researched diseases in the world today, so we can be hopeful of changes.

Q: My neighbor's mother is on some special experimental drug for treating Alzheimer's. What is that?

A: It could be one of several, such as Cognex or Aricept. These drugs developed out of the greatest success in research: following the actual progression of Alzheimer's disease and trying to find ways to intervene in that process.

Neurotransmitters are the chemical messengers of the brain that begin to fail in their duties as the disease develops and progresses. We don't know why this occurs, but researchers are now able to replicate those chemicals so that people can be treated by supplying them with the missing or depleted chemical messengers. This supplementation can help people to recover their cognitive losses or at least to improve them somewhat.

So far, although no silver bullet has yet been found to supply the magical cure-all, promising studies are being conducted in various nationwide exploratory programs. Your neighbor's mother is probably involved in one of these.

Those who wish to participate in such programs should ask their doctors whether they can get into one. Family members should know, however, that such programs may not supply the whole answer. For every one of these programs, some people are helped a great deal, some a little, some not at all. For others the side effects of the drugs may be too extensive for them to continue. Give this range of response, it is often worth considering being enrolled in a drug testing program if one is available.

We may now start to look forward to successful interventions in the process of degeneration, since so much research is going into studying the process. Although we still do not know why people get Alzheimer's, we do know increasingly more about how the disease progresses.

Q: Is it true that you only know for sure that someone has Alzheimer's after they're dead?

A: Yes, but then again, no.

What you've heard is the often stated medical opinion that only autopsy establishes that a person had Alzheimer's, since we don't know for sure until we see the evidence of plaques and tangles in the brain. However, even that may not be as definitive as your doctor tells you. Here's why.

In 1987 a major world conference on Alzheimer's disease was held in Germany. International experts on the disease came together to examine some of the biggest problems involved in its exploration. The major problems a decade later are still the same ones, although medical science may be reluctant to admit this publicly.

Basically, there are three major categories of problems. The first is that, as we have stated, we do not know what normal aging is, let alone abnormal aging. Therefore, we have a dilemma: If all aging brains have some plaques and tangles—and they do—how many are too many? Answer: We really don't know.

The second problem is that pathologists, on whom we rely at

present for the final confirmation of Alzheimer's given in autopsy, are often working from different sets of criteria. For example, since many of the brains being autopsied have already been designated with Alzheimer's disease, there is a tendency for the pathologist to assume that any sign of degeneration must be due to Alzheimer's. This has created a circularity in the research that may actually obscure or skew the studies.

The third problem is that the relationship between neuropathology and clinical manifestation of Alzheimer's is not clearly established. For example, pathologists have designated people who never manifested dementia in life as having dementia, based on the state of the aging brain at death. The brain shows extreme degeneration, but the person when alive did not behave as if demented. This may sound strange, but most doctors who work in brain injury rehabilitation will confirm that extent of injury and the manifestation of impairment in life do not run parallel. People retain their own mysteries when it comes to functioning in life, and some do better than others for no discernible medical reason.

Perhaps it comes down to the mystery of individuality.

One very recent discovery made by scientists at the University of Pennsylvania Medical Center are plaque-like lesions in brains affected by Alzheimer's disease involving a previously unidentified protein. Such lesions are rare or absent in other neurodegenerative diseases. Possibly this might be a confirmed marker for Alzheimer's disease and may also give new clues as to its origins.

Q: Since doctors don't yet know what causes Alzheimer's disease, what are some of their theories, at least?

A: Over the past twenty years, several different theories have arisen and been dismissed, sometimes to recur again. These theories include aluminum, genetics, toxins, life events, and lifestyle factors.

Q: Is it true that aluminum causes Alzheimer's?

A: The aluminum theory suggests that aluminum in the brain causes disease and that removing the aluminum removes the dementia. This theory dropped into disfavor for a few years, only to reappear in 1991 as a contender.

There has been supporting evidence for this school of thought, but not definitively enough to ensure an answer for everyone with Alzheimer's. Evidence suggests that people with Alzheimer's may be particularly sensitive to the accumulation of toxic metals. Iron has also been questioned as a cause, as have mercury and copper, though these are less well known than the aluminum theory.

Human beings are exposed to aluminum much more than most people realize. Aluminum is used in cookware, and aluminum salts are used in the cleansing of our public water supplies. Aluminum also appears naturally in rivers and streams. It is the main ingredient in most deodorants, and it is used in the containers of nearly all canned soft drinks and a great deal of food packaging.

It is also true that populations exposed to high amounts of aluminum, in certain areas of Canada and in Wales, have statistically much higher incidences of Alzheimer's, but that still does not prove that aluminum is the only candidate as a cause. It could be merely a trigger in people already predisposed toward developing Alzheimer's because of some other factor.

Q: My grandmother had Alzheimer's just before she died, and now my aunt has been diagnosed. Does this mean I stand a good chance of getting it?

A: There is a genetic theory of Alzheimer's, which may or may not involve heredity. A hereditary disease runs in the family, whereas a genetically caused disease is due to prenatal factors. Neither has really been established as a clear cause of Alzheimer's, although there are indistinct links.

Of course you're worried. That's understandable. But you need to know there is very little statistical support for a genetic or hereditary cause of Alzheimer's for most people.

You have probably heard about the "Alzheimer's gene," but so far research has not found one—not really. There is a genetic basis for certain chromosome defects and mutations associated with some early-onset Alzheimer's. Problems found in chromosomes 14, 19, and 21 have been individually linked with familial forms of dementia in a few families; these defects seem responsible for the appearance of early dementia, beginning in a person's thirties.

If you have one of these chromosome problems, you should worry. Clearly your grandmother did not have early-onset Alzheimer's, however, but the usual after-sixty-five type of Alzheimer's. Probably the same is true of your aunt. In that case, as a member of a family in which Alzheimer's has appeared in more than one generation, you have only an 8 percent chance of developing Alzheimer's, which is pretty low.

As a nonmedical person with common sense, I ask why we don't call these rare chromosome-specific dementias by different names, such as chromosome 14 dementia, chromosome 19 dementia, and so on, instead of lumping them in with Alzheimer's disease of people aged sixty-five and over, which is apparently dementia caused by different reasons.

Q: I read there's a special gene that shows you will develop Alzheimer's. What is it?

A: You may have read about the apoE gene theory of detecting predisposition toward Alzheimer's disease. All human beings are born with one of three variations of the apoE gene, and researchers at Duke University have found that those with a variation known as apoE4 seem to have a high risk of developing Alzheimer's. Does this sound bad for you if you have the apoE4 gene? Well, take a closer look at the research.

The team carried out genetic testing on sixty-seven people who had been diagnosed with probable Alzheimer's disease. They found out that forty-three of them had the apoE4 variant of the gene. The team also carried out the usual brain autopsy, looking for the telltale plaques and tangles of alleged Alzheimer's disease. Fourteen of those tested did not have the apoE4 gene present but did have the plaques and tangles. An additional ten also did not have the gene and also did not show plaques and tangles although they had shown dementia-like behavior in life.

This means there *might* be a 65 percent chance that the apoE4 genetic variation *could* be an indicator of the possible development of Alzheimer's disease, if healthy people of sixty-five and over do *not* also have the apoE4 genetic variant in the same ratio.

That is a pretty indefinite statement, so I would suggest not to worry for now. The reality is that too little testing of healthy people has taken place for us to even guess what health looks like, and finding factors like these in diseased people is vague at best.

There is some significant new research from the National Institute on Aging, following through the apoE4 gene discovery. The latest results state that people who inherit two apoE4 genes—one from the mother and one from the father—are eight times more likely to develop Alzheimer's than those who inherit two of the more common apoE3 gene.

Q: We've heard you can get treatment for Alzheimer's in Germany using drugs you can't get in the United States. Would you suggest we take our mother there? We're certainly willing to do what it takes.

A: I wouldn't. You could spend all her money and all your funds chasing desperately from one rumor of treatment to another. While it is good to remain hopeful, families would be wise never to become too gullible.

It's unlikely that a cure in another country has not already been checked out in the United States. If there has been a breakthrough, information can be found in your own hometown. You can do all your research in advance of making any such decision by using the Internet and checking out all the sources that are undoubtedly available through your local library.

Arm yourself with as much knowledge as possible before putting your mother into the hands of doctors you've only heard about by rumor. Good and successful research is published widely. It is also unlikely that only one doctor has the answer, especially if that doctor is charging a lot of money and has not shared the results of his or her research.

That said, it is also true that there is, or has been, a medical bias in this country against exploring possible help from the fields of alternative medicine—usually called complementary medicine in other countries. One big reason is that most research in this country is funded by pharmaceutical companies looking for a marketable drug, a situation that can theoretically result in bias.

This is why you will find approaches to Alzheimer's from herbal and homeopathic medicine among M.D.s in Britain, France, and Germany. I suggest looking into those by reading extensively in professional publications, such as the prestigious British medical journal *Lancet*. Most of those discoveries are available in the United States. See also chapter 8 on Help from Alternative Medicine.

It is unlikely that there will be a one-pointed cure for Alzheimer's disease, since it seems to have many complex aspects to its evolution.

Q: Is Alzheimer's the only dementia?

A: No, there are many dementias and many conditions that cause dementia, either temporary or permanent. Apart from the large number of other conditions that present a dementia-like appearance, including depression, drug reactions, thyroid problems, nutritional deficiencies, brain tumors, hydrocephalus, and head injuries, other medical dementias include:

- multi-infarct dementia, caused by many small strokes and vascular problems
- dementia resulting from Parkinson's disease
- Pick's disease
- Creutzfeldt-Jakob disease
- Korsakoff's syndrome, a dementia resulting from alcohol abuse
- AIDS dementia, which is becoming much more common. AIDS is showing up more and more among people over sixty-five.

Q: Suppose they do find that Alzheimer's is a genetically caused disease. What does this mean?

A: There is a tendency to regard the mysteries of a disease as basically solved once it is identified as "genetically linked." But we cannot say for sure whether a genetic tendency toward Alzheimer's means that a person will or will not develop the disease.

We do know this about some diseases and genetics. For example, in the case of the notorious Huntington's chorea, any child carrying the gene will undoubtedly develop the disease. However, the study of genetics is still new and in many areas unexplored. We have no clear idea about the statistical meaning of genetics when it comes to Alzheimer's disease. Although anyone who has a parent with Alzheimer's will probably worry about getting the disease, there is little statistical evidence to support that fear.

We also cannot eradicate the other factors that play their part—the triggering events, the emotional factors, the environmental factors, injury or previous illness, and so on. Even if we can prove that all forms of Alzheimer's disease are genetically linked, we cannot eliminate the other triggers without considerable research. Currently, we are not yet able to claim that Alzheimer's is always genetically linked.

Insurance actuaries have developed a list of factors that predict the possibility of major accident or disease. Accumulate enough of these factors and you become *statistically at risk* to fall prey to a serious medical condition or a serious accident; yet, nowhere will this appear on your medical record. How much do such factors affect your chance of developing Alzheimer's?

In the literature of Alzheimer's, there has been very little exploration of this; yet, Alzheimer families have anecdotal accounts of common events that seem to be triggers.

Until we know more, we cannot say that Alzheimer's disease does not come about as a psychospiritual crisis, the collapse of the immune system due to overwhelming life conditions. No one in the medical establishment suggests this at the moment, but the role of trauma in the onset of major manifestations of Alzheimer's needs to be researched, as do other sociological biodata, which have been neglected so far.

Q: If it isn't genetics and it isn't aluminum, what else could cause Alzheimer's?

A: The other factors that researchers feel may yield some secrets of this disease include the following:

1. *Environment.* In an age when we have many questions about the state of the environment and the extraordinary levels of pollution most of us live with today, it is obvious that any system failure as vast as Alzheimer's must bring up the examination of whether the environment plays a part in this disease.
2. *The slow virus theory.* A number of challenging diseases, such as multiple sclerosis and some cancers, are now being associated with slow viruses. We know fairly little about slow viruses, how they work and how to stop them from working, but some researchers suggest a connection.
3. *Head injuries.* Studies have shown that a significant number of people who manifest Alzheimer's disease have also suffered major head injuries at some point during their lives. The statistical evidence shows that people with

Alzheimer's have indeed suffered serious head injuries three-and-a-half times more often than people who don't get Alzheimer's. However, we don't know what this figure really means and what the role of injury is in Alzheimer's development.

4. *Psychiatric medications.* This is a little-explored aspect of Alzheimer's as yet, but a study from the Mayo Clinic showed that as many as one-third of patients with Alzheimer's had undergone psychiatric treatment and, therefore, had presumably been treated with psychiatric medications.

   Another linked question: Is there any relationship between the very high number of elderly women with Alzheimer's and the widespread prescription of drugs like barbiturates, tranquilizers, and antidepressants for women during the 1950s and 1960s, which often continued for thirty years or more? Since it is drug companies that fund most drug research, we may never see this factor being explored.

5. *Trauma.* The most common anecdotal story in the onset of Alzheimer's disease is its association with a trauma. It is as if the body's immune system collapses and Alzheimer's overwhelms the individual, leading to a rapid onset of serious dementia. Not enough studies have been carried out into this aspect of Alzheimer's, but the question is there.

Among the biggest traumas that come to the elderly are loss of a spouse and relocation, often forced by circumstance. Other traumas include loss of abilities through age or illness, loss of friends, and loss of previous lifestyle caused by the inability to maintain it due to personal changes.

Early childhood trauma, loss, or deprivation may be another factor. One might question the relationship between the figure that one in four women are sexually molested in childhood and the significantly higher numbers of women who have Alzheimer's, as compared with men. Few studies, however, are being conducted in this area.

The number of factors linked with Alzheimer's disease suggests that its cause may be multifaceted. Unfortunately, most research is not multifaceted. Instead, it is significantly pointed toward drug research and toward a single-factor cause.

Q: Will there be a treatment for Alzheimer's soon?

A: We can certainly hope so, since so many researchers are exploring avenues of treatment.

Some promising signs of help are on the horizon. A few years ago there was excitement about a drug called tetrahydroaminoacridine, THA for short, now often called tacrine and marketed as Cognex. It seemed to bring about memory improvement.

Despite its initial promise, it was observed to cause severe liver damage and later some of the early promising test results were called into question. In 1991, a drug advisory panel recommended to the Food and Drug Administration that the drug be discontinued as an Alzheimer treatment.

Widespread outcry resulted. The families of Alzheimer patients were pushing for more freedom in getting experimental treatments on the market. The drug is now being tested in a new series of nationwide experimental programs. It is now admitted that the original claims of vast improvement have not materialized and that the rate of improvement, where it exists, may be around 10 percent.

Anecdotally, some families report great improvement in their sick family member; others report some improvement; still others report no improvement or problems from side effects that necessitated quitting the treatment. Cognex has a hotline available to support families, with nurses to answer queries—an excellent idea, although families have occasionally reported experiencing pressure to continue the drug. Cognex sales representatives frequent Alzheimer's seminars, and families need to remember that sales reps are not impartial information sources.

Following the aluminum theory, some researchers are working with a drug called desferrioxamine, credited with removing aluminum from the body. However, since other researchers are claiming that aluminum was never a significant issue but only a contaminant in laboratory testing, we don't know how this research will affect treatment.

Other researchers are excited about drugs that may help to supply the missing chemical messenger in the brain, acetylcholine. In 1976 researchers were already connecting low levels of choline acetyltransferase (CAT) with Alzheimer's disease. This research has a number of followers, each trying to isolate the right drug or chemical that will bring acetylcholine levels back to normal. We can expect to see several developments in this particular area since no one is actually disputing this theory of treating Alzheimer's.

Other research is looking into the role of a protein called beta amyloid, which is found in great excess in the brains and bodies of people with Alzheimer's disease. It remains to be established what the actual significance of this protein is. At first, researchers thought they would be able to use the presence of beta amyloid as a way of testing the presence of Alzheimer's and coming up with a definitive diagnosis. However, more recently, teams of researchers at Case Western Reserve University in Cleveland, Ohio, led by Steven G. Younkin, have established that this protein is widely found throughout the cells of both healthy people and people with Alzheimer's. More of it is found in Alzheimer's patients, but it is not known whether this is a symptom or a cause. Since some researchers suspect the excess of this protein may actually be one of the pathological processes in Alzheimer's, they are developing anti–beta amyloid drugs to see if they can halt or decrease Alzheimer's, or even reverse its effects.

An interesting development in this particular line of inquiry is the discovery that substance P, a natural brain hormone discovered in 1931, may prevent induced brain damage in rats.

Researchers are trying to demonstrate whether substance P could be used to fight Alzheimer's.

Some exploration of transplanting fetal brain cells into deteriorated areas of the brain to see if the brain can be revitalized is being conducted. This has so far been applied only to cases of Parkinson's disease, with some good results, but many questions remain. One man who could barely walk is back at work, but others have shown more ambiguous results. This is still being research, and there are major ethical questions to be considered. Other researchers are looking at whether artificially increasing blood supplies to affected areas of the brain might bring about that same revitalization.

All of these are exciting and, we must hope, groundbreaking explorations that could lead to the breakthrough we all want to see, the one that will overcome Alzheimer's disease.

Q: Since there's no cure for Alzheimer's, does this mean there's nothing we can do for someone suffering with this illness?

A: No. In fact, in our frantic search for the silver bullet that will magically slay the werewolf of dementia, we often overlook other ways in which people with Alzheimer's could be helped considerably in the here and now.

For example, few therapists and counselors work with people with Alzheimer's, and yet the fear levels surrounding this disease are tremendous. Talking about what is happening can be helpful for people, but I suspect this seldom happens because of societal prejudice toward the impaired and the brain-damaged. Therapists can be just as influenced by such biases as anyone else, and I suspect that's the reason why so few have looked into helping people with Alzheimer's.

A lot of therapy deals with the primal family relationships, and people with Alzheimer's often have an excellent memory for childhood and early life events. Instead of turning readily to the use of harmful drugs, less invasive therapy could bring about peace, relaxation, and resolution and reduce bizarre behavior.

People with Alzheimer's can be helped with the following:

1. *Exercise.* They can and do follow interesting exercise, whether yoga, tai chi, or just movement and walking.
2. *Bodywork.* This population, starved for touch and knotted up with tensions, responds well to touch.
3. *Play therapy.* Many people with Alzheimer's have a deep willingness to play and explore, but guidance is needed for them since they can rarely initiate play. In these activities, people can find triggers that enable them to talk about their anxieties or fears or sadnesses.
4. *Relaxation.* Since fear and apprehension are such constants among people dealing with dementia, these people also suffer from extreme tension. They are often willing to follow relaxation exercises—stretching, breathing, even simple guided imagery—and they benefit greatly from these. They also respond well to relaxation brought about by use of essential oils and aromatherapy.
5. *Music therapy.* Music reaches into the heart of a person with Alzheimer's and brings light and pleasure. Classical, ethnic, New Age, popular music all work well.
6. *Talk therapy.* Far from losing their memories, people with Alzheimer's actually seem to be overwhelmed by them. It is true they are often confused about which part of the time continuum they are living in, but they are usually not confused about their struggles for parental love and acceptance. Therefore, all the material for talk therapy is available, and real emotional changes come about that then affect daily life experiences.

These simple things could make significant breakthroughs in dealing with the behaviors that are so often the cause of other problems. We might find that people then do better with the disease.

As well as looking for drugs, let us encourage research into finding ways to bring these people peace and resolution. If we fix only on a cure, certain types of healing—which have nothing to do with cure—may never take place. If we feel the only success is cure, all our Alzheimer relationships have to be seen as failures. Instead, we need to develop the kind of understanding that has developed around other diseases, such as cancer and AIDS.

It's important to realize that a person may still die of a disease and yet experience healing of the heart and spirit. People with Alzheimer's need our love and our acceptance. They need most of all to know that we accept they are as vulnerable and unprotected as children, that they feel as scared, and that they can feel as magical as children.

Perhaps no other disease depends so totally on the caregiver. Alzheimer's imprisons people. Just as small children cannot really escape their home, people with Alzheimer's cannot escape their disease, though some try. We can make their disease an endless cruel sentencing, or we can help them find peaceful resolution.

Family Crisis, Alzheimer Style

Whatever joy there is in this world, all comes from desiring others to be happy. Whatever suffering there is in this world, all comes from desiring myself to be happy.

—Shantideva

In my years spent working with families dealing with dementia, I've noticed how reluctant families often are to get help. I suspect this is partly because Alzheimer's can go on for so long and because dealing with it seems endless. There are so few definite answers, and a long struggle can pull families apart. Families rarely prepare themselves for the ordeal, and often years are wasted while people make mistakes and take wrong turns. This chapter will explore ways in which families might reduce the struggle and anxiety of their ordeal by learning early on what is needed and how they can help each other.

Q: Why is Alzheimer's different for families than, say, cancer?

A: This is a disease of mental function rather than of physical body, therefore it can cause endless dysfunction in the family itself. Alzheimer's is extremely variable, as varied as people are, and this is not true of most diseases.

Alzheimer's asks of families that they learn new ways to make a successful relationship with the person who has the illness and that they become willing to let go of the past picture of who the sick person once was. This is why it is very important for all family members to tackle the Alzheimer problem together from the outset, if they can.

Q: Does Alzheimer's make families crazy, or are they already that way?

A: Families deal with disease the way they deal with life. Because Alzheimer's is an often subtle and infinitely variable disease, it tends to bring about crisis even in the best-organized and healthiest of families. This is because the beginnings of the disease involve loss of ability to function, rather than specific symptoms needing specific treatment. It is a disease of behaviors.

In families with unhealthy interaction patterns, Alzheimer's disease becomes a new battleground. Members of the family will fight with each other and even with the person who is sick.

Q: I just feel the situation is all so meaningless. Is there any way to find some meaning or purpose in this horrible disease?

A: Rather than ask for meaning in the disease, perhaps it helps to look for meaning in how to cope. Ask yourself, "How am I being asked to grow?"

Even for healthy families, this disease brings many moments of crisis. A series of difficult decisions must be made, even though the family may lack sufficient information to make informed choices. Often, they are working without support, without help, and without education in Alzheimer's disease and its ramifications.

Learning how to do all this is what brings about growth. It doesn't matter that we didn't ask for that growth and don't want it, it can still be ours.

Q: I feel like I've lost my mother altogether since she's developed Alzheimer's. How can I get through the next few years without going crazy?

A: You're facing a major crisis by being forced to revise your relationship with your mother. This hits many family members hard. It's one of the great ordeals in Alzheimer's.

A son or daughter must face the gradual loss of a parent; the adult child becomes parent to the mother or father. It is hard for any child to take on a parental role toward a parent figure. It goes against family history with its psychic life and all the complications of parent-child relationships. Plus, Alzheimer's brings additional fears to the children of its victims. They wonder if this is a picture of their own future. It is a meeting place of loss, fear, and yearning.

A spouse, on the other hand, has to adjust to loss of partnership while at the same time gradually taking on care of someone who has childlike needs.

The only way to make sense of this ordeal, or to make it meaningful, is to learn how to cope well. That means getting the support that you need for yourself. Learn what you need to know, go to a support group, take stress management classes, and give yourself time off.

Try to work at creating a new relationship with your mother. She needs your love and your help and, if you can learn to sit still with her, she may turn out to have things to share that you don't yet know about. No matter what your previous relationship was, your new one will need a lot of loving touch, time to be together, and your willingness to come to where your mother is.

If she was a good mother to you, you will already have learned how to be nurturing from her. If she wasn't all that great, this is the time to heal that lack by becoming something like a good mother to her.

Q: Isn't it codependent to become a caregiver, and isn't it bad to be codependent?

A: It isn't codependent to become a good caregiver, only to become an overwhelmed, overworked, overachieving caregiver who can't do the job well or lovingly.

Many families today are tied to unhealthy patterns of relating due to a variety of sociocultural reasons, so we can expect to find them entangled in the Alzheimer world, too. There, the care of the sick person becomes a desperately embattled business. Siblings are likely to find old issues revive, with unanswered needs and suppressed angers surfacing.

A child who seldom received nurturing care from a parent will find it harder than most to become that same parent's parent figure. Family members who have not learned to respect and cherish each other are not likely to treat the sick person with respect, appropriate attention, and acceptance. Unhealthy rivalries and wars may arise again, all fought in the shadow of one of the most demanding of illnesses.

Society itself is dysfunctional when it comes to Alzheimer's disease. Society projects all its deepest fears upon this disease: the terror of being dependent on others, of losing control of life, of becoming an object of pity, and of losing one's mind. Therefore, through these projections, society sets up Alzheimer's as the disease no one can cope with.

It isn't true. People *can* learn to cope well.

The battles of Alzheimer's can also be subtle. Merely because your family is not actually fighting does not mean you have escaped dysfunctional patterns. It is always good to examine your own capacities and to revise them where necessary.

Q: How do you know if a family is being dysfunctional in its caregiving?

A: To know this, it is useful to look for certain patterns. The following are among the signs of unhealthy family attitudes around Alzheimer's.

Denial

Q: My father won't admit there's anything wrong with my step-mother. He says she's fine, yet she has serious memory problems, she dresses weirdly these days, and she doesn't seem to be able to do anything around the house like she used to. I think she might have Alzheimer's. How can I get him to face it?

A: It's not unusual for people to deny the presence of a problem, especially an older person who may have been brought up to believe in keeping one's troubles to oneself and not sharing them, even with other family members.

Think about why your father is in denial. Is this his life pattern? Is he overprotective of your stepmother? Does he really not notice? Or is he too scared to admit what's going on? All of these are possible.

Write down all your observations so that you have your documentation at hand and wait for a quiet moment in which to raise the subject. Be very clear that there is no blaming or judgment in what you say, just a real desire to help.

If he feels he can trust you and has your support and respect, he may be able to share this with you. If he is still not ready, you may have to be a more subtle helper and do what you can without his admission.

You can't break down a wall of denial. Only feeling safe will allow your father to lower his defenses.

Q: My sister lives with our mother, who has Alzheimer's. I know it's hard for her, but I worry when I hear her being so mean to our mother. She says our mother could manage if she wanted to, that she's just faking it so other people have to look after her.

A: It sounds as if your sister needs more help in several directions: more time off, more education about Alzheimer's, and possibly some kind of counseling if she is unable to accept your mother's illness or if she has long-held emotional issues with your mother.

In some families, members may deny to each other that the situation is as serious as it really is, often treating the afflicted person as though he or she could choose to manage better. The sick family member is blamed for the illness. The sick person gets accused of not trying hard enough, being too needy, or deliberately behaving badly when showing symptoms of the disease. People use the person's symptoms as a way of proving they are behaving badly. This attitude may represent family anger or ignorance.

Family members may find elaborate explanations to deny the existence of the illness. One family, for example, talked about "Mother's nerves," not her Alzheimer's disease.

A family may deride or castigate the sick family member for exhibiting the symptoms of illness: "Ma, I told you that already!" as if the person did not have short-term memory problems. "She doesn't even wash properly anymore—it's disgusting!" as if the inability to take care of personal hygiene were a deliberate choice.

These are all aspects of denial, and they have their roots in different parts of the caregivers' own personal issues, issues with the sick family member, and sometimes the caregiver's issues with the disease itself. Dealing with them takes a lot of personal integrity and commitment to coping better and to being a better caregiver by exploring personal issues of fear, loss, and anger.

Q: I told my husband that the doctor said he had Alzheimer's disease and he yelled at me. He shouted, "There's nothing wrong with me. You're the crazy one!" How can I make him believe the doctor?

A: Your husband's response is called denial. You cannot make him believe anyone right now.

Denial has a purpose and it gives us valuable information about a person. It tells us this person is not yet ready to face the truth, that he or she is probably feeling great fear.

Your job is to gradually take over the responsibilities that your husband can't manage anymore and at the same time give him what support you can. When and if he begins to feel safer, then he might be ready to hear you and his doctor. Nothing will shake a denier, so family members need not worry that the truth will hurt. The impaired person will brush it off.

Anger

Q: My grandmother shouts at my grandfather when he gets muddled up. She thinks he's just doing stuff on purpose to make her mad, but his doctor says he has Alzheimer's. I'd like to help, but I don't know how.

A: Your grandmother may be frightened by your grandfather's behavior or she may simply not love him anymore and be overwhelmed at having to cope with his illness on top of everything else.

Either way, she and he need help. Anger arising in families coping with Alzheimer's takes many forms, and your grandmother's reaction is a common one. In other situations, we find that family members become enraged with each other over differing opinions on treatment and plans for the sick person. They get mad at each other's behavior. They are unable to let go of their demands on each other or forgive each other's shortcomings in coping with the illness. Sometimes, as in your grandmother's case, this rage is directed at the person who is sick, either as obvious abuse or more subtly as constant criticism, irritation, and demeaning treatment.

Despair

Q: Every morning when I wake up, I remember my husband, Hal, is sick with Alzheimer's disease, and then I just want to lie there and not even let the day start. I feel like I'm sinking down so low I'm going to drown. What can I do?

A: You may have gotten yourself trapped into thinking that your problems won't be over until Hal is dead. Although your problems may have started with his illness, you can begin to find ways to deal with them right now. You don't have to wait until he's dead before you can find ways to feel better.

It's natural to have a grief reaction to learning that your husband has Alzheimer's disease. But if this feeling has deepened into a lingering despair, this is an unhealthy response that will steal your life and energy.

You can begin to learn different ways to cope. While there is currently no effective treatment or cure for Alzheimer's, there are still many ways to make life feel worthwhile and emotionally valuable, even in the midst of the crisis of living with a loved one who is seriously ill. Or, let's be really honest here, maybe you did not love your husband enough to feel you can go through this ordeal with him. Only you know the answer to that.

Either way, you can change things for yourself, starting today. You can begin to find the best ways of dealing with this situation. Alzheimer's is lived both by the person who has it and by you, the caregiver. When the caregiver sinks into despair, as much as we may sympathize, the situation is not being dealt with. Your continuing sense of despair suggests that you may be resisting the personal change needed to bring about a new way of relating to the situation.

Start by making a list of your needs and another list of your problems. Be very specific. The problem is not so much that your husband has Alzheimer's disease, but what the disease is doing to *your* life. For example, perhaps you don't get enough sleep, enough time off, or enough privacy. Perhaps you feel guilty because you wish he were dead or you're scared of the future. Perhaps you're angry at him for getting this disease and spoiling your lives. These are all normal and understandable feelings.

Be really honest as you make your list. Once you're done, start to go through the list and make decisions about how you are going to meet your needs. For example, get someone to sleep over in your home so that you can sleep at night; seek counseling for your emotional issues, and so on.

What you can't fix right now, cross off your list for another day. Make another list of good things you can do for yourself right now—breathing deeply, soaking in the tub. These are not small and irrelevant things. They are ways to increase the quality of your life.

If you're too overwhelmed to even start on a list, drag yourself to a support group, a counselor, your minister, rabbi, mullah, monk, or priest. If you can't get out of the house, make a phone call. If you can't get to the phone, pray, even if you don't know who you're praying to. Just say, "I'm really in trouble and I need help. Please send help." Despair is a stagnant situation. As soon as you start to do anything, however small, you begin to shift that despair.

Blame

Q: *I've got two brothers and we're all trying to deal with Pop's Alzheimer's. They get mad at me and mad at him and I don't know what to do. Help!*

A: The blaming family is commonly found in the Alzheimer world. Instead of uniting to form a battle strategy to deal with Alzheimer's, working out family approaches, and reaching a consensus, the family breaks apart. This division often continues for years after the crisis.

There are usually two reasons why this goes on; you will recognize which applies most to your situation. It can happen because there has been a previous pattern of divisiveness, but it is also often caused by a family's inability to face loss, fear, and the pressures of role changing, as well as their terror of the disease itself. Family members blame each other instead of confronting their own feelings about the disease.

Perhaps this is what is happening with your family. See if all three of you can agree to talk things over following my plan for the Family Council (see section later in this chapter), which sets firm limits on family members' participation in a meeting. If you can't get agreement, find a mediator. If that doesn't work, try to reach agreement on one person as the executive caregiver.

Avoidance

Q: *Isn't it kinder not to tell someone he or she has Alzheimer's disease? What's the point? It would just scare the person.*

A: We see this avoidance in family members refusing to talk about the disease with the person who has it: "I couldn't possibly

63

tell my husband he has Alzheimer's. It would really upset him and I don't want to hurt him."

This may sound like consideration, but it is actually the speaker's inability to reach out to the other in a painful situation. It echoes the old habit of secrecy around cancer, and it condemns the real victim to loneliness and fear.

Believe me, the person with the disease has already known for years that something awful was wrong. We do that person no favor by denying the opportunity to speak about what is happening. Often, bizarre and violent behaviors are triggered by a family's refusal to break the silence around Alzheimer's.

Once the truth is out, everyone can help support each other, including the person with Alzheimer's, who will need to be reminded from time to time that he or she is ill.

Q: When should I tell my wife she has Alzheimer's? Sometimes she catches hold of my hands and begs me to say what's wrong with her. I don't know what to do.

A: Your wife is more than ready to know what's wrong with her, and you won't hurt her with this truth, even though it's a hard one. It will probably be a relief for her. When people don't know they have Alzheimer's but they do know there's something wrong, they blame themselves for being stupid or crazy. Hearing she is ill will let her off those hooks and allow the two of you to become closer. All studies show that people would rather hear the truth about their illnesses even when the news is bad. It will not hurt her, and it isn't cruel to tell her. The devastating thing about Alzheimer's is having it, not *hearing* that you have it.

Q: What should I say when my mother (who has Alzheimer's) says she's always forgetting things? I usually say something like, "Oh, well, I forget things, too." Is that right?

A: When someone says, "I forget so much," it may not be as kind as it seems to gloss over it by saying, "Oh, well, we all forget things. I'm always forgetting things myself."

There is a major difference between the global forgetfulness of Alzheimer's and ordinary memory glitches. It might be more reassuring to show understanding and empathy by saying something like, "It must be hard to forget so much, but it's not your fault, you know. You have an illness that causes you to forget things."

Usually, people are surprisingly accepting of such news, even relieved by it. Of course, I'm assuming you have already talked to your mother about the fact that she has Alzheimer's.

Q: *My grandmother has had Alzheimer's for years now. She lives in a home and we hardly ever go to see her anymore. Is there any point? She doesn't know us.*

A: Oh, but don't *you* know *her*? It must be really inconvenient that she's slipped in her memory of faces, but she didn't do it to hurt you. It's one of the symptoms of her illness.

If you don't love her anymore, who will? Does being family stop when a member gets impaired? And if you do love your grandmother, how is she ever going to know that if you never go to see her?

From years of observing people visited in long-term care, I know that you can fill up the heart of a person whose memory has holes in it. Staff see the difference in those elders who have loving families visit them—they are richer, fuller, and more substantial than those who never have visitors.

In other words, it does matter and makes a difference.

Q: *What should I do to make my visits to my aunt more meaningful or pleasant for her? She's got serious dementia and she doesn't always know me, but I've always been fond of her and I'd like to go on seeing her.*

A: Good for you; even if your aunt can't really express it to you, your visits matter. When you visit, greet her in a loving way and also introduce yourself, identifying your relationship. This is her cue that you're related.

Take her gifts that she appreciates—something to eat or flowers, if she likes them. Plan some activity to ensure a good visit—maybe looking at a family photo album, listening to a tape of music she enjoys, or another activity you might do together. If she can go out, take her for a walk or drive, with a stop at an ice cream parlor, somewhere that the two of you can relax. Keep within her energy level—probably a short walk and a short ice cream stop, but possibly a longer drive.

Good planning plus patience during the visit will be the key to successful time together. Remember also how important a loving touch is; sit near your aunt, perhaps with your arm around her. Often, old people in care homes sit in isolation all the time, especially if they are in wheelchairs. You might bring her some scented hand lotion and give her a soothing hand massage, or brush her hair if she would like that.

Don't be too busy around her to actually give her your undivided attention, something that often happens when family members feel awkward about visiting a sick relative.

Q: Do you think it's demeaning to give an Alzheimer's patient a soft toy, like a fluffy stuffed animal or a doll?

A: It's never demeaning to meet someone's needs at the level of their functioning. It's only demeaning to assume all people with Alzheimer's want or can or must relate to toys. If a person would enjoy the comfort of such a possession, if it would be soothing or emotionally fulfilling for that person, I think it's fine to give one.

Often, it is caregivers who have to overcome their own demands for higher functioning from those who are deeply impaired. People with Alzheimer's do not have to perform to our standards. We have to become sensitive to their needs and capacities and respond appropriately.

Q: My sister says she can't bear to see our mother, who's now living in a care home because she has Alzheimer's. She says it's too painful. Well, it's painful for me, too. How can I make my sister visit more?

A: Apparently you can't. It's very hard when one member of the family—and that seems to be you in this case—becomes the designated caregiver. It's hurtful when family members do not come to see the person who has Alzheimer's. It's also a burden for the caregiver.

I don't know your sister or what's bothering her. It may be selfishness or emotional immaturity in being unwilling to deal with the reality of your mother's illness, or it may indicate serious emotional maladjustment to all the issues of old age, disease, death, and loss.

I suggest that you give some thought to how you can deal with this so you get more peace. If you can't change your sister, maybe you have to change yourself and work on letting go of your anger with her. That doesn't mean she's right or that she deserves such consideration from you. But *you* deserve that much. Use the energy that may be absorbed in anger or resentment for something more constructive.

The reality is that your sister doesn't get off scot-free—not really. She will carry an inner burden for everything she evades. You can work off all your issues while being with your mother and being her caregiver. Consider some counseling to help you get to that sense of resolution.

Q: We're five brothers and sisters, and four of us are closely involved with looking after our dad. Our oldest brother keeps away, but he sends money when we need it. How can we get him more involved?

A: It sounds as if he is as involved as he can manage for now and that sending money is his way of meeting your dad's needs.

Don't let differences in commitment divide your family; try to forgive the failings of your brother. I'm sure you're wise enough to know that you will lose by holding on to resentment.

Q: *We still visit my mother on a regular basis now that she's in a nursing home. She's real confused most of the time, but I want my children to know she still matters to us all. My husband thinks it's hard on them and that I shouldn't take them to visit her. What do you think?*

A: The family that avoids visits is avoiding in the short term its feelings of pain, loss, and helplessness, but all of these feelings tend to catch up in the long run. Guilt over unfulfilled duties and omissions of love lasts a lifetime and often creates the dread of being similarly abandoned in need or old age.

If we demonstrate that our elderly are not valued, we set ourselves up in time to also be valueless to our family members. If we show that love and caring are always valuable, we teach our children something worthwhile about loving.

By visiting your mother, you're giving your children great training for life.

The Designated Caregiver Syndrome

Q: *Why is it always me who has to look after my mother? I have brothers and sisters, but you'd think I was an only child when it comes to taking care of our mother.*

A: It's probably you because you let it be you. Families often quietly designate one member to do the caregiving. There is no pattern to this designation. Sometimes it will be an unmarried daughter, or more rarely an unmarried son.

However, it may also be one particular family member, whether married or not, with children or not. This choice is obviously connected with previously assumed family roles. Perhaps you volunteered in the past to carry out caregiver roles. Perhaps you just did not resist being put into the role.

It's time to tell everyone how you want things to be different. As you express clearly what you need, you may find others taking up more helpful roles, but you have to be specific about what you want for yourself, about the time you want, about the exact nature of the help you need.

Q: I live nearest to my mother, so my sisters expect me to look after her, even though I have three kids to raise by myself. I wouldn't mind quite so much if they didn't question every single thing I do. They've got plenty of opinions but they don't help at all. Any suggestions?

A: However the selection takes place, the designated caregiver often gets to do all the caregiving with no practical family help other than long-distance telephone calls offering opinions, advice, and criticism. That person becomes virtually deserted by the rest of the family, except when major decisions are involved. Even then, they may not get support from the family but only input.

Obviously you are stuck in this classic family dilemma. You don't detail the issues, but I wonder if one of them is money— your mother's money. Make sure you don't get into money struggles with your sisters. It can be a good idea to call in a lawyer and have your mother's finances tied up neatly and cleanly. Otherwise, you could be accused of financial abuse of your mother. Remember that you should be the financial conservator to handle her money. Even sharing a joint account does not keep you safe from accusations of financial abuse.

If it really is the day-to-day decisions that your sisters question, either suggest they take over your mother's care themselves or tell them that you make the decisions. One suggestion is to tell your sisters you have to leave town for a few days (you think up some reason) and so they have to take over. This usually settles this kind of interference.

See if you can get the family to talk everything over and allow delegation of decisions. If they can't come to town, you can do it by conference call.

Another question to consider is, how were your relationships with your sisters before all this happened? Is this part of a family pattern? Could therapy help you handle this better for your own well-being?

Q: I look after my wife all the time and I love her very much. I'd never put her away anywhere. But I hardly ever get to sleep through the night anymore and it's real hard to take care of the house.

I have two daughters but they're pretty busy so I thought maybe I should get a woman in to help so I could get a little break. My daughters said, "Oh Daddy, don't," so I didn't, but my daughters didn't help any more than before.

A: You could wait for your daughters to come around, but you might be dead before then. Here's a hint: The person who does the work gets to choose the rules. Your daughters are being selfish and unkind. They may also be scared you're going to replace their mother with this helper or have an affair with her.

Can you stand up to them and yet also discuss these matters in a nonthreatening way? Tell them gently but firmly that you are dying by degrees and that they must either help you every day or you will get help in the house.

Then hire the helper as soon as possible. You deserve help, and so does your wife.

Q: My brother doesn't believe our father is as sick as he really is with Alzheimer's. He lives in another state and calls Pop on the phone every week or so. Pop sounds fine on the phone and makes up a bunch of stuff and none of it's true. As soon as my brother rings off, Pop doesn't even know he called. The result of all this is my brother refuses to help us at all. How can I get him to understand?

A: You'd be surprised how often this happens. People with Alzheimer's may be able to cover up and put on a good social front in a telephone conversation or a brief face-to-face chat.

If family members never visit, they have no means of checking out the situation. It is not uncommon for them then to suggest that the caregiver is exaggerating the problems.

Insist that your brother come to relieve you of duty for a weekend or a week. If proving a point is your aim, a weekend will usually do it. One weekend spent with a person who has Alzheimer's disease is Alzheimer boot camp, a thorough basic training in what the caregiver's life is really like.

This has set many a family straight and ensured that at least they do not emotionally sabotage the caregiver's work by denying the need for it.

Q: *I belong to a large family, but no one helps me with my aunt. I can't go on without help.*

A: Set limits, as hard as this can be. Family members must be asked for definite commitments to allow you time off. Don't give in on this, tough it out.

If your family members are geographically close, ask them for a daily break of some kind. If they are far away, then relief every six months is not unreasonable. If your family resists helping, then hire the help you need. If your money is short, ask your family to help pay for hired help.

Q: *Where can I find someone to help me look after my husband? We have no family to help us.*

A: Do as much outreach as possible into the community for additional help. Use all possible day respite programs. Ask your friends for help. Hire a few hours of help a week if you possibly can. Use the full range of suggestions in this book.

The Family Council

There could be many ways to hold a Family Council, from having a weekend retreat together to holding a telephone conference. Its form is not as important as the agreements made.

If many family members are involved, it might even be a good idea to outline preliminary agreements on how decisions are to be made—by consensus, by concession, by majority vote—so that the actual council session will be useful.

If very few members are involved, this should not be necessary. Mainly, the focus should be on achieving the best care under the circumstances, with the proviso that the best care is that which best meets the needs of the person who has Alzheimer's.

With a very troubled family, it might be very useful to have an outsider to mediate the meeting, so that family members can be called to order if necessary.

The most productive council session does the following:
- does not allow personal attacks;
- does not develop into battles of willpower;
- stays concentrated on the practical issues;
- lists the practical issues and deals with them one by one;
- writes down results with everyone's agreement;
- sets a plan in place.

Even though these are not easy to achieve, some agreed action must be in place before the session closes.

I have explored the form and agenda of the family council more fully in my book *The Alzheimer's Sourcebook for Caregivers*, and therefore will say here only that it is most important for family members to respect each other's views and feelings. They do not have to agree with each other, but an attempt at mutual understanding is important.

Individuals in the same family can feel they have experienced an entirely different kind of family life from other members, and this is their emotional reality. Others cannot argue them out of it, nor should they, and neither can they argue them into it, which is often hard for them to accept.

Family action plans must be made around what members will commit in terms of time, money, and effort. They cannot be constructed around what members feel that other members ought to commit. That way, fights erupt between family members while the person with Alzheimer's gets left out as far as his or her own needs are concerned.

In order to create workable plans, everyone has to make and meet his or her own commitments. If another family member avoids such commitment, as reprehensible as that may be, that gap needs to be filled by those who will commit.

Q: I go and stay with my parents every weekend. My father's been sick in bed for four years now and I live a hundred miles from them. My sister isn't even working and doesn't do anything for them. She also lives a hundred miles away. I yelled at her to make her do more. Now she won't even speak to me on the phone. How can I make her do her share?

A: You can't. Neither can you make plans for your parents that count on you making her do her share.

As unfair as it seems, some people manage to do more and better than others and so they end up being the ones who do what needs to be done.

Do people like your sister get off free? No, not at all. My observations over the past ten years tell me that those who fail to help family members in need never get off the hook from failure, guilt, and pain. Those who do what they can, on the other hand, are able to come to peace and fulfillment because of it.

You can command only your part of the journey. Better practice letting go of your need to control your sister so you can enrich your own life with that energy. She clearly has her own psychic journey—maybe she just can't deal with her parents' needs and weaknesses, maybe there are reasons she is angry at them, or maybe there are things in her life you are unaware of that prevent her being able to help. Maybe she is selfish. Or just plain irresponsible. Whatever it is, you cannot make her behave.

Perhaps this is also the time to accept that you cannot do your parents' own journey. You can walk with them and help them, but they have their own personal journey of age, need, illness, and death from which you cannot save them.

So, look after yourself and do what you can, then let go of the rest.

Chapter 5

Education and Acceptance: The Secret of Alzheimer Success

We are not helpless as we experience painful or distressing situations if we can creatively respond to those circumstances with dignity and courage.
— Christine Longacre
in *Facing Death and Finding Hope*

What you probably most need to know when dealing with Alzheimer's is how to cope with the problems peculiar to it. Most of these problems are not really medical. Many of them are behavioral, as are many of the solutions.

Until you understand two things, you are in constant trouble. First, Alzheimer's demands behavior changes of everyone living with the disease—everyone except the person who has the disease. The sick person can no longer be expected to conform to other people's expectations. Second, everyone "does" Alzheimer's disease in his or her own way.

Families who do not accept these two truths, who fight, deny, or ignore the changes they must undergo, will only lock themselves into a losing battle of demanding that the person with Alzheimer's change, adapt, or somehow get retrained.

This chapter will explore ways in which education and acceptance can lead to Alzheimer success.

Q: Our doctor told us what to expect as our mother's Alzheimer's disease goes on. It sounds pretty grim. Is that what we have to look forward to—someone who'll be crazy with anger, who'll run away and get lost, who'll never let us sleep?

A: There is a big difference between medical outlines of Alzheimer's and the reality of living with your mother. It's a pity doctors don't do a better job but sometimes dwell on the negatives. The caregiving can indeed be hard, but that doesn't mean it's the end of the world.

First, you are already an expert in this area. You know your mother. You probably already know what upsets her, what pleases her, and what enrages her. You know what she can do, and you know that her capacity to manage may be greatly reduced at times. You probably know how to bribe, persuade, and cajole her successfully to get your way.

So you are already an expert in one area of Alzheimer's. Your first piece of education is to acknowledge that you are an expert. No doctor, nurse, or social worker knows your mother like you do, and that's what counts. Your mother doesn't turn into a stranger with symptoms. She's your mother with a disease.

You might try writing down the things that you already know about dealing with your mother's Alzheimer's. In fact, it would be very educational to keep a daily journal. It will help you to get a grip on things and it will be a valuable record. If other people become involved in caring for your mother, your notes will help them to know what works, what usually happens in certain situations, and how to deal with events. Such a journal need not be elaborate. You do not have to be a writer. Just jot things down. You will probably become aware of many more things as you do this.

It is also useful to learn as much as you can about the disease itself. This may not be easy, since there is little real incontrovertible information available on this disease and you probably already know more than most people. But you can learn its typical behaviors, and this will help you and your family to avoid battles you cannot win.

Q: Sometimes my husband can do everything for himself and yet other days he can't manage to dress himself and seems really confused. What's going on?

A: The symptoms of Alzheimer's can vary literally from day to day, usually according to the general condition of the person, either in physical or emotional terms.

So, if your husband is more confused or less able to dress himself on a particular day, it probably means he is having some other problem that is causing him to fail in his general functioning. For example, if he feels unwell, has a cold or a touch of flu, or is coming down with an infection, it may show in the dysfunction you mention, rather than in the symptoms you might expect. It is hard for a person with dementia to recognize and communicate that he feels unwell. Instead, the communication is acted out in behavioral problems and incapacity.

Alzheimer's itself does not suddenly get worse, unless some very damaging trauma has taken place, such as an accident, general anesthesia, an injury, or a loss. It usually worsens gradually, so a sudden overnight change may indicate a health problem. Schedule a visit with your doctor, who can check for infections or other developing conditions.

Q: My mother lives with me. She has Alzheimer's and sometimes she has "accidents" because she doesn't get to the bathroom in time. This always seems to happen when I need her to hurry up. Is she really doing this to spite me?

A: No, she isn't doing it on purpose, even though it feels that way to you. Alzheimer's disease takes away the kind of capacity that would allow her to plot against you.

My guess is you're overstressed and overtired and perhaps lonely or lacking the other support you need. To make life easier on yourself, you need to be able to step back sometimes and be an impartial observer. That is not always easy, especially if you are angry or overworked. However, you will be better able to deal with the problems of caregiving if you can maintain your role as an observer.

To be the impartial observer, you need to know who you are as a caregiver, especially your emotional fragilities and your personal stress reactions. Again, a journal will allow you to learn about yourself as a caregiver and enable you to watch out for the ways in which you get caught up in the stress of the situation.

There is no need to blame yourself; we are all human and we all have our shortcomings as caregivers, especially when we are tired or upset. Self-knowledge will help you make the appropriate allowances for yourself, and you will find it easier to look on your mother's failings kindly.

Get an early start instead of trying to hurry your mother. Stress is the trouble for both of you. She feels your urgency, and she is reacting with her own stress problems.

Q: How can we find out more about Alzheimer's?

A: As part of your education about this disease, read the whole problem-solving chapter (chapter 7), which covers many of the intricacies of dealing with Alzheimer's that often only caregivers know about. Another way to learn more is to attend as many workshops, training classes, and seminars as you can find.

There is, unfortunately, a dearth of practical knowledge being given out in workshops. Too many programs deal with new medical research and the latest drug testing experiments, which do not offer families the kind of relief they most need. Attend such workshops anyway, and be prepared to ask questions. If you have particular requests, make a note of them before the workshop or seminar so that you will not forget or be too intimidated to ask.

Don't forget to check out your local branch of the Alzheimer's Association and find out where support groups meet (see appendix B). Support groups are probably the most important source of information for you. Other caregivers know who the good doctors are, ways of dealing with problems, and your area's resources.

They also know the daily grind and its hardships in a way that only caregivers can. It can bring you relief and a sense of peace just to be with people who know this situation. You never have to feel ashamed among caregivers, because they understand what you're going through and they always have an encouraging word.

Other parts of your education will include research into financial and legal issues. A husband and wife with shared resources should look into safeguarding their assets, ensuring that power of attorney is taken care of, and doing their estate planning for the future.

Unfortunately, until the health care system in the United States is revised considerably, Alzheimer's disease can bankrupt a family. The right kind of financial planning can help to avoid some of this. Some couples have divorced simply so that they could protect their assets.

There are now a number of ways around such situations, but it is a highly specialized area with legalities and financial details varying considerably from state to state. Therefore, it is very important that you consult an expert in this field. Usually that will be a lawyer with expertise in elder law and estate planning, with special reference to issues of providing for long-term health care.

Be sure the person you see really is an expert in these issues. Check out references and recommendations from local organizations—for example, the American Association of Retired Persons (AARP), your local Agency on Aging, elder services, and senior centers. When you do find someone who is recommended, do not be shy about asking what experience that person has had in such estate planning. You want someone who has dealt with hundreds of clients needing this service, not a handful. Be ruthless about your questions because this professional can make or mar your future financial well-being. Many experts suggest that you do not allow this person also to handle investing your funds.

If your planning is done prior to a diagnosis of Alzheimer's, your family member might still be eligible for long-term care insurance. You obviously cannot get such insurance after the diagnosis of Alzheimer's, but you might get it before any suspicions you have about your family member are confirmed. Be extremely careful to check what any such insurance actually covers.

Do not take out policies on the advice of your insurance agent alone. Take time to think things over and ask an independent expert to look over the policy. Ordinary health insurance will cover normal hospitalization even if Medicare does not; very few other policies really cover long-term care although many claim to do so. The national headquarters of AARP reports that many spurious long-term care insurance policies avoid paying out just when you need them to.

Alzheimer's disease is covered by very few policies, so be suspicious and do not let yourself be talked into anything. Your local senior center, senior services agency, and AARP branch can probably help you with this matter.

If you are facing the possibility of placing a family member into care, don't assume that you need insurance or have to pay cash down to the verge of ruin. It is not true that you cannot keep your family member in a place in which he or she is already comfortable after resources have been spent down and Medicare takes over. Many reputable care facilities are part of a federal aid program that allows them to keep a resident at this point. Such facilities get federal grants in return for being part of the program. You can get this information in advance and choose your facility accordingly, picking one that guarantees your relative can stay once Medicare kicks in.

Do not imagine that such residents are treated any differently from those who are paying full rates. They are not. State regulations ensure that every resident is treated with the same respect and gets the same care and attention. If this were not so, the institution could lose its license for infringement of state and federal laws. Remember that money does not buy certainty when it comes to good care, so do not be too attached to having to pay for everything yourself.

Q: I'm looking after my husband myself right now and I intend to do this as long as I can. But one day I may have to place him in care if this gets to be too much for me. How do I find a good place?

A: Learn about the range of care facilities in your part of the world. Read chapter 11 on placing someone in care so that you know well ahead of time what your possible alternatives are. Not everyone with advanced Alzheimer's disease has to be placed in a skilled nursing facility. In fact, most people with Alzheimer's do better in a smaller, more homelike environment that gives both care and companionship in a supportive way. Look around at small home care residences so that you have a good idea of other choices well ahead of the need to make a decision.

Visit care facilities until you find one you like. That way, you won't be caught by surprise or rushed into a decision you may regret. Don't be discouraged that few places are really what you want. Remember, you need only one.

Q: How do I know when my wife needs more care? Is there something I should watch for that would tell me it was time?

A: Learn about the possible course of this disease, while also acknowledging that it can vary greatly. That way, you will recognize certain changes as they happen.

For example, you will notice when vision changes cause a person to be unable to center on a chair or toilet seat; be ready to help act as a guide. You will be alerted then that you should probably be around your relative when he or she goes up and down stairs, just to keep an eye on safety hazards.

As to making that decision for placement, it really depends on the two of you. When your wife needs more than you can give, that's when you need to find her other care. If you can't get that care in your home, then you need to find a facility where she can get that care.

To know when she needs more than you can give, be realistic

about yourself. Are you getting enough sleep, enough time off? Are you physically, emotionally, and mentally able to cope? Are you suffering from stress? Becoming ill? At the end of your tether? Get help. Consider placement. Placement is *not* failure. It is the only way to ensure that someone gets twenty-four-hour care.

Q: Yesterday I had to tell my wife six times to switch off the light. Finally I did it myself. Why won't she do what I tell her?

A: Mainly because she probably doesn't understand what you're telling her. Many people with Alzheimer's have trouble connecting nouns with their meaning. They simply don't remember what, for example, the word *switch* means. If you can point to what you're talking about, then she may understand. Remember, this is a symptom of her illness. She's not doing it to annoy you.

Knowing what is happening in the course of the disease will help you be much more accepting. For example, when you begin to realize that your wife is no longer connecting words with their meaning, you will not get angry when your questions or commands are not carried through.

Such education keeps you sane. Another good way to stay sane is by educating yourself about good caregiving and about caring for yourself as a caregiver. This is very important. The biggest problem for caregivers is the drop in their own health due to lack of stress management. This is often the most neglected aspect of caregiving. Caregivers put themselves last, but unfortunately this only guarantees that they will not be effective in their task.

Q: Everyone says you're supposed to manage stress, but how?

A: Stress management classes are often offered at senior centers, in recognition of the stresses of old age. Do not dismiss these classes thinking you cannot learn anything useful. You can.

Take exercise classes, especially gentle exercises like yoga and tai chi. Learn about what your diet should consist of as you age. All these things will be part of your education for survival.

Other ways of educating yourself could include learning how to communicate better, especially if your relationships with your family members are not going well. If you are an elder yourself, you might have learned ways of communicating, or not communicating, that do not serve you well anymore. Relearning such habits and finding better ways to do things and talk about things will form part of your network of help.

Q: I help look after my uncle, who's got dementia. My aunt wants to keep him home even when he's dying. I want to help her but I'm scared of him dying. Can anyone help me?

A: They certainly can. Fortunately, there has been a whole development of help around death and dying. Today, no one who is helping a dying person has to approach this process without support.

First, you have probably heard of a hospice program at your local hospital. This is a program designed to help people who want to die in their own homes. Nurses and hospice volunteers will give practical help and support to you and your aunt throughout the process.

Second, the library carries books on the subject of death and dying. Don't be scared to read these, since they are not frightening or morbid—far from it. In fact, they will help you to understand that death is natural and that it is something we will all do one day. You've probably heard the saying, "You don't get out of life alive!"

Here is a short list of must-reads: Elisabeth Kübler-Ross's books *Death and Dying* and *Questions on Death and Dying*; Stephen Levine's *Who Dies?*; and Sogyal Rinpoche's *Tibetan Book of Living and Dying*, which has some excellent advice on sitting with the dying.

If you feel you know nothing about the process of death and dying, consider attending workshops or training courses on the subject. Most hospice organizations offer these from time to time. You might even consider volunteering so that you will feel more comfortable when your uncle's time comes.

The main thing you need to know is that the typical Alzheimer's death is quiet and peaceful and with little struggle.

Q: My doctor says I should get counseling to help me deal better with my husband's Alzheimer's. Does he think I'm crazy?

A: Probably not. I imagine your doctor would like you to have more help and support in helping yourself through this difficult time. Getting counseling is a normal way to get such help these days. Perhaps you believe that only sick people go to counseling, but actually it is a very healthy choice.

Be open to learning from experts how to cope better with life. Life with Alzheimer's has many burdens, so don't scorn getting help, guidance, or a chance to talk things over.

Talking things over with a professional may help you to see a situation more clearly. In the old days, family members provided this kind of support. Now, many people do not even have a minister, priest, or rabbi to discuss life difficulties with, yet life has become increasingly more complex. Allow yourself to get that extra help and input where it can do most good.

Q: How do you know when you need help from a therapist?

A: Here's a suggestion. Take a look at this list:
1. I feel trapped and helpless.
2. I am tense and unhappy every day.
3. I can't face the day when I wake up.
4. I can't sleep.
5. I feel so guilty every time I get angry.
6. I don't know who to turn to.
7. I don't think I can go on much longer.

Did you answer "yes" to any of those statements? If so, you should seek help from counseling.

Q: How do you find a good counselor?

A: To find a good counselor, ask your local senior services agency. Ask your doctor for references. Check out any local counseling offices or services. They are usually listed in the Yellow Pages under Counseling or Therapy.

It may take a few attempts to find the person you feel most comfortable with, but you will benefit from this effort. It is up to you to work out with your therapist how often you will go. Counseling does not have to be long-term or expensive. You will probably find that your health insurance covers at least part of the payment.

Q: Is it true that Alzheimer's interferes with medications?

A: The problem is not that it interferes, but that it obscures medications. Medications work differently on people with dementia.

Once a person is manifesting Alzheimer's disease, the norms for body response change, becoming variable and highly individual. Drugs are never tested on people with dementias, except in the case of Alzheimer-specific drugs. This means that no one can say how a particular drug will affect a person who has Alzheimer's disease. Side effects that might be minor in reasonably healthy people could be devastating in those with Alzheimer's.

Caregivers must do two important things. First, ask your doctor what the side effects of any new medication are, according to the manufacturer. If your doctor does not know, or seems to be shrugging you off with vague reassurances, ask your doctor for a copy of the printed information on side effects supplied by the manufacturer. This way you know what to look out for. This is very important since your relative probably will not be able to tell you, "I feel sick," or "My vision has gone blurry." You will have to watch for unusual behavior from your relative. Keep daily notes after any change of medication so that you have a documentation of new behaviors or troubling developments. Do not accept that these changes are not due to the medication. Ask your doctor to try withdrawing the medication to see whether behavior becomes normal again.

The second thing you can do to safeguard your relative is to demand a change, reduction, or cessation of medication if drastic changes occur.

Extremely little is known about the effects of medication on people with Alzheimer's, so you are the resident expert on its effects on your relative. Keep notes and be firm.

Q: We're a family of five siblings trying to look after both our parents with Alzheimer's. We're devastated by this and we're driving each other crazy with arguing and fighting over the best way to do things. Before we all kill each other, do you have any suggestions to help us?

A: I suspect you're all reeling from the shock and terror of this double disaster, so let me take you through a process that can be helpful.

Perhaps the most important thing is that you all accept that there really is no perfect, no absolutely right, no unarguable way to deal with this disease.

Try to use the outline for a Family Council (see chapter 4) to come to an agreement on an action plan. Also encourage each of your siblings to confront his or her own feelings about Alzheimer's itself, since I suspect that terror of the disease may be one of the chief causes of dysfunction for all of you.

This is very important for the future of the family. Make no mistake: this is a disease that divides families forever, not a temporary crisis soon over. A crisis can bring everyone closer together for a while. However, a long-term struggle allows each person to behave according to personal patterns of behavior.

Q: Is there anything going on in people with Alzheimer's, or are they just empty, not there?

A: That's the big lie about people with Alzheimer's: they are regarded as shells, as vegetables. It's just not true. It's simply that we look away and don't bother to listen anymore.

In old age comes a deep reworking of the primary issues of love, abandonment, wounding, and healing. This is why so many older people are preoccupied with their early lives. It is a normal part of maturation and reconciliation in life, of coming to peace.

It is exactly the same for the person with Alzheimer's, who is also deeply involved in those primary relationships, still trying to work them through and reach peace within. The main difference is that the person with Alzheimer's has often actually forgotten that those parent figures are dead, that this is some entirely different year from the one they are thinking about.

So when the person with Alzheimer's reveals that he or she actually expects his mother (long dead) to come home that night, the caregiver often focuses on the time error caused by dementia. We can help by concentrating instead on the concerns the person is expressing. We can focus on the feelings about the parent and the unresolved issues being discussed.

We can help most of all by becoming an ideally loving parent figure so that the longing for love and safety and acceptance—common to all human beings—can be fulfilled in the here and now. By giving unconditional love now, we help heal the wounds of the past.

Talking
Alzheimer Talk

Words are one way we build bridges to reach each other, but every communication between human beings is immensely complex. Even when two people start with the same language, the same set of inner assumptions, and the best of intentions, their words can become more like barriers than bridges. For those with Alzheimer's, this art of communication can become a freeform chaos in which everyone gets lost.

One can see why. Good communication relies on good brain structure to carry it all. The system that connects thought, ideas, concepts, speech, and utterance needs to have all its mechanisms in working order. In Alzheimer's, the brain chemistry itself is unable to support this communication, and the system falters. Memory cannot carry thoughts through. Words cannot remain attached to their meaning. Speech may not express the thought within. Feelings may trigger words that do not communicate their sense.

From all this chaos within, the person with Alzheimer's tries to reach out to others, to cross the broken bridge.

Q: I notice my husband starts sentences, then kind of drifts off as if he's forgotten what he was thinking. He gets very frustrated sometimes and hits his head with his hand really hard. How can I help him when he feels this way?

A: One thing you can do is to show that you notice, understand, and empathize with his dilemma. Don't be afraid to reveal that you know. He knows! It will help him feel less alone.

Caregivers often see that it becomes hard for the person with Alzheimer's to formulate and express complex thoughts. This difficulty shows up in many ways: the person mishears or misinterprets what is said; the meaning of words may be disconnected from their sound; even if the person hears accurately, he or she may find it impossible to construct a logical reply; even if the capacity to think cognitively is present, the speech center of the brain may not obey the person's wishes and the wrong words may emerge, as happens to stroke victims.

Or, as in your husband's case, he can't hold a thought long enough to finish his sentence.

Q: *Why is it hard for people with Alzheimer's to say what they want or tell you what's bothering them?*

A: In Alzheimer's, many obstacles lead to roadblocks in normal communication. We could assume the messenger system of the brain becomes like a damaged computer, with parts of the program missing. Without the structure supplied by these missing bits of programming, the person is left trying to make sense of a world that seems crazy.

When you're aware that someone is having this difficulty, you might say, "I can see this is frustrating for you. I'm sorry," and indicate that you're willing to wait patiently. This helps to remove the emotional pressure.

It's usual for a person with dementia to keep forgetting he has an illness and to blame himself for being stupid or crazy. Loss of control of life causes high levels of fear and anxiety.

Don't be afraid to broach these subjects. Just airing them can do much to relieve stress.

Q: My aunt keeps repeating the same things over and over, like some broken record. None of it makes much sense. Does Alzheimer's make people nuts or what?

A: There is one single most important thing to remember about all this: the person with Alzheimer's disease is not crazy, however strange the behaviors. Therefore, every communication has a purpose, and our task as caregivers is to find out what that is. No words or actions are meaningless, even what sounds like nonsense, or continuous repetition of the same words. Everything is intended to express a feeling, to show a need, to give information, or to get a response. As caregivers, we need to remind ourselves constantly that Alzheimer-afflicted people are trying to understand everyday life, just as we are.

The difference is that an essential part of their information system has been disabled. It is like being a stranger in a strange land, not understanding the customs or speaking the language very well. Instead, everything that is familiar and loved about life becomes strange, unknown, and therefore often frightening. Even the people we love become strangers, since we may not be able to name them correctly or place them in context.

My guess is that your aunt is lonely, frightened, and feeling unloved and unappreciated. Repetition of the same words might be her way of trying to comfort herself.

The more you learn about Alzheimer's, the better able you will be to help or bring some comfort to your aunt in this difficult situation.

Q: I work in an Alzheimer's care unit and we get people there who do strange things or act out. I'm wondering how we can help them.

A: Again, if we accept that all behaviors are meaningful, then we are left to ask ourselves what the meaning of this behavior is.

As caregivers, we also need to ask: What unmet needs are being expressed by this behavior? Acting out becomes a symbolic portrayal of their truth. People with this disease are constantly acting out their needs and their feelings within a fractured brain structure. As caregivers we often witness apparently bizarre behavior or are confronted with peculiar demands. Stressed-out caregivers often fall into blaming the person at this point, simply because the complexities of communication are too overwhelming, added to everything else that has to be taken care of.

This happens in care institutions just as it does at home, for the same reason: overworked, underrewarded caregivers under stress. In institutions, we often label such behaviors "difficult" and such people as "combative." The trouble is, labeling doesn't solve much. Only decoding the behavior can help us to find solutions that help the resident.

Q: Is there some special way you should talk to someone who's demented? How do you know they understand what you're saying to them?

A: Speak kindly and with great attention. Use sentences that are clear and simple in a voice that is soft and kind. Sharp and hurried tones will only cause agitation, nervousness, and dysfunction. Complexity causes intellectual overload, which will bring about a distress response—perhaps rage, tears, anxiety, or extreme slowness and inability to do tasks that normally can be done.

It is a good idea to speak on the same level as the person, both literally so you can be face to face, and figuratively so that you express ideas in a way that can be easily absorbed. But do not patronize. Just because people have Alzheimer's disease does not mean they are insensitive or stupid. They are simply functionally impaired, and they are often quite aware of their own and other people's feelings.

Because of dysfunction, they may sometimes say things that we would consider inappropriate and hurtful, like, "Oh, you're fat," but this is due to the loss of societal inhibitors that were taught when they were young.

Approach the person from the front so you can be seen. Surprises are not welcome in the world of dementia. Speak clearly, give plenty of time for the person to respond, and avoid memory questions. You may find it useful to be sure you have the person's attention by gently placing your hand on his or her arm, hand, or shoulder and being sure you make eye contact. Alzheimer's patients often spend periods of time in altered consciousness, and they need to be gently brought back into the here and now if they are "away."

Many caregivers think it appropriate to ask a person with severe memory problems all kinds of questions involving the use of memory. Memory capacity can vary from day to day, and some days will be worse than others. That is why on some days the person with Alzheimer's will remember you, some days she won't. It is just Alzheimer weather.

The past is a murky country for the person with Alzheimer's, and the future has often become unimaginable, but the present is always with us. Therefore, we can always rely on the present to be part of our communication, a part the afflicted person can fully share.

Q: Should I tell my neighbor who has Alzheimer's who I am every time we meet? It feels so silly.

A: I know it does, but not as silly as your neighbor feels not knowing you and yet sensing that you know her. So, yes, it's a great courtesy to introduce yourself each and every time.

Here's an example of how not to do it: "You remember me, don't you? Can you tell me what my name is? Do you remember what we did last week? We really enjoyed ourselves. Don't tell me you've forgotten already!"

This would be much less distressing rephrased as, "Hello, Irene, I'm your neighbor Mary. I live just across the road there and we had such a good walk together last week. Maybe you feel like going on a walk with me now?"

Relatives, too, should learn this new social skill of introducing themselves. This will help to remove some of their distress when their family member cannot get their names right.

Q: My father calls me by his younger brother's name. That uncle is dead now. Should I correct him when he doesn't know me?

A: I suggest you see how it goes when you do correct your dad. People with dementia tend to set their own level of functioning. If your father is feeling that it's 1926, he probably won't understand that you are not his younger brother. In his reality, there was no you back then. I'll bet you look like his brother.

Often family members feel hurt or bewildered when their names are forgotten or they are confused with members of a previous generation. However, there is a certain logic to what is going on. The person with dementia does not remember what year this is and therefore tends to inhabit whatever year he or she is thinking about or remembering.

People who are in a separate "time zone" like this usually follow a logical process of thinking about the people who inhabited that time zone with them. Therefore, people born after that time are fitted into the memory zone in a logical way: they become the uncles, aunts, brothers, and sisters of the past, often following their family resemblance. Rather than rejecting the person, this is actually an acknowledgment of their closeness and connection; it's just that the facts are wrong.

Q: My husband gets so confused when he dresses in the morning. Sometimes he gets really angry when he can't manage and tries to hit me. How can I get us through this chore without these tantrums?

A: As people become more deeply impaired by Alzheimer's, they find it harder to complete the tasks of daily living. Since they know they are impaired, they become frustrated and upset. At this point, your husband may need constant verbal cueing to do things like get dressed, take a shower, and so on.

The main thing to remember about any such cueing is that it must be done one step at a time. Memory failure means your husband cannot keep a number of actions in mind. Give one instruction at a time and point to the objects you name: "Here, Jerry, why don't you put on this sock? That's it. That's great. Now this one. Good. Now here's your sneaker. And, let's see, here's the other one."

Constant conversational accompaniment can be very soothing. Never give orders, always make suggestions, and never insist. Always back off if there is a problem and return to it in a few moments. Never try to hurry your husband through step-by-step procedures. Hurry causes dysfunction.

If he's getting clothes upside down—sleeves are especially confusing—or can't tie his shoelaces, help out physically in an understated way.

Maybe he needs simpler clothes, such as slip-on shoes and sweatsuits rather than lace-up shoes or button-down shirts. Be willing to experiment. Buy some items and offer them without much comment. Often such changes are met with no reaction or even acknowledgment. Have his clothes laid out for him, since making choices can be very hard for a person with dementia. If he resists a procedure, ask yourself if it is necessary and drop it if it is not.

Q: My wife has Alzheimer's. We still try to do all the things we used to do. She always enjoyed doing the shopping before but now she often gets upset in the supermarket. I wonder if I should go shopping without her.

A: It is probably overwhelming to her now—too many choices, too many reminders of what she can't do, maybe too many people. Yes, I suggest that you take over.

Going shopping is a rational process. It involves selection, thought, planning, and choice-making, all of which become hard, if not impossible, in Alzheimer's. Save both of you the trouble.

Q: When I ask my husband what he'd like to eat, he gets agitated. Why is this?

A: Again, the problem is selection and choice-making. Probably your husband does not remember what he'd like to eat. Instead, offer him a choice of two items you can show him. This gives him the power to choose without stressing his memory.

The danger of referring to absent objects is that you have no way of knowing for sure that you are understood. Since you know his tastes by now, why not just serve up meals without consultation?

Q: As a caregiver, how do you get someone with Alzheimer's to do what you want? I notice my husband doesn't respond well to being confronted.

A: Few of us do, and certainly confrontation is not something that works well in Alzheimer's. The rational process is lacking, plus so much fear and apprehension are present in the person with dementia that confrontation tends to be overwhelming.

As a caregiver, you will find that mastering the arts of cajoling, bribery, manipulation, and gentle persuasion will be effective, just as they are for the mother of a young child. These arts will be a cornerstone of your communication practices with the person who has Alzheimer's disease.

Other helpful management tools: suggest and lead, instead of giving orders; allow plenty of time; and show lots of love and humor.

Q: My husband keeps asking when I'm going to take him to his mother's. The problem is she has been dead for many years. Should I tell him that? I did once and he cried. I felt terrible.

A: Often caregivers come up against questions that seem to demand hard or painful answers. While it's important to be truthful, it's also important to understand the real question.

A man who asks for his mother, especially if he does this often, may really be talking about the desire to be mothered. That is the desire you need to concentrate on. Therefore, if his question is, "When are you taking me to my mother's?" it could be answered in that time-honored response of mothers, "Not now, honey."

If he actually demands to know whether his mother is alive, he must be told the truth and, if necessary, allowed to mourn. After all, it is not inappropriate for a man to weep for the loss of his mother. It simply means he is feeling very orphaned at that moment, and grief is appropriate. We cannot take away the real human journey of the person with Alzheimer's, one that will inevitably involve dealing with losses. When you are asked difficult questions that lead to problems, you will soon learn how to evade, concur, or be conversationally noncommittal about them. This may cause dilemmas for you at first. Most of us want honesty in our communication with others. We do not feel good about lying, rightly so. However, in dementia, we are often presented with situations that bring up specific issues in which blatant literal honesty causes great pain and confusion. For example, a weeping eighty-year-old woman says, "Why hasn't my mother been to see me? I haven't seen her for a long time."

What is the point of telling a human being who desperately needs mothering that her mother is dead? This is neither necessary, relevant, nor kind, nor does it meet her needs. A much more appropriate, relevant, and kind approach would be to say sympathetically, "Are you missing your mother now?" or "Are you feeling lonely?"

If such a question brings tears, you have not failed. It is an honest, human response. Console the person and be loving, without guilt. Sometimes caregivers mistakenly feel it is their duty to protect people with dementia from all reality, including pain and sadness and reminders of their losses. These are part of the human journey.

Q: In our care unit, we're supposed to keep people oriented to reality. So, what's the best thing to do when someone's talking as if this was the Second World War or they're living back home with their parents seventy years ago? Are we really supposed to get them to admit this is now? And how do we do it?

A: Ah yes, reality orientation—a profoundly misunderstood concept! Reality orientation was a program initiated in a Veterans Administration hospital in order to keep temporarily and mildly confused patients oriented to their surroundings. It was never meant for—and neither is it successful for—use with the permanently and profoundly demented.

Caregivers of people with dementia must respect their reality. It is not the duty of the afflicted to live in our reality. It is only the inexperienced, rigid, or unkind caregiver who rams so-called real facts down the throats of lonely, frightened old people.

Another often ignored fact is that no one can forcibly change the reality of a person with Alzheimer's. Very often, the demented person knows emotionally exactly what is needed and will not be distracted from that need. The displaced one wants to go home, even if he is sitting in his own home. The one who feels useless and unwanted wants to cook dinner or clean up the house, which is no longer hers and may not even exist anymore. The frightened, lonely one wants Mother. Just as small children want only what they want, with a deep emotional intensity, so too do those with Alzheimer's. Reality orientation is not possible with them, on the whole. It is meaningless because they are expressing their feelings, not concerns about facts.

Q: Why do people who are demented tell the same stories over and over?

A: That's not unknown behavior even among those who don't have dementia! However, people mainly do it because they have a story to tell and a need to tell it.

It is not memory loss that causes a person to repeat a story, except in a superficial sense. Something—pain, fear, insecurity— may keep triggering a particular memory. If caregivers address this by responding to the person's feelings, the person will no longer need to repeat the story. It will be exorcised, leaving the person free—we must hope—to return to more pleasant memories.

Many individuals stick with their happy memories. One elderly woman who lived in a nursing home gave birth to a baby every night. She was overcome with joy and triumph and her happiness was so clear to the staff that eventually everyone joined in. Staff would look in on her and say, "How's that baby coming, Grace?"

Q: What about people who make up stories about their past that aren't true?

A: We could give this a psychiatric label and talk about delusion and hallucination. However, this does not seem to get us anywhere, except to give us a vocabulary. A vocabulary does not give us the tools to deal with the person. Since Alzheimer's is not defined as mental illness, the language of mental illness is not appropriate.

People being besieged by Alzheimer's go through great pain, fear, and loss at various stages. This is especially true in care institutions, where most fable-makers seem to be found. We can regard the stories as a coping device, a way of making the unbearable bearable, even a way of making a new life when the real one did not fulfill many needs.

Some professionals feel that people with dementia should have their invented realities adjusted to factual life, forcibly if necessary. It can never be done successfully, however. It seems far more humane and considerate simply to accept that this is the way their reality is.

People with dementia have two needs: a need for us to respect the adult in them and a need to honor the child that may gradually emerge.

Q: Is it true that most people with dementia stop being able to talk?

A: Not necessarily, although it is true that language is likely to fail gradually. I have heard of one man who early on apparently forgot how to speak, but what we usually see is language becoming more fractured. For example, the person starts using names less often—something that may happen in the very early phases.

Nouns used abstractly may not be connected to their meaning anymore. The person may not be able to find the words needed. "Could you buy me one of those. . . you know . . . small and I had two in my refrigerator but now there's only one," turns out to be a request for lamb chops. (Incidentally, the caregiver understood this message.)

Language connections may be lost, either because of memory failure—the inability to hold a sentence in mind so it can be completed—or because of brain dysfunction, so that rational thoughts literally cannot go through the right neural pathways. Sentences may stay uncompleted or become very convoluted as the person goes on determinedly but cannot get quite the right words and phrases out. For example, "I think that something soon will happen that is terrible if something soon is not done," was Hilda's way of saying, "I urgently need to get to the bathroom."

Gradually, the impaired person may say less and less and seem to be further and further away. This "awayness," which is certainly some kind of altered state, often goes on for longer and longer periods. None of us knows where these people "go to," but we do know, from brain studies, that people with Alzheimer's dream much more than most. This sense of interior preoccupation is often found in the later stages of the disease. Those so affected give the impression, not of being the living dead, but of being the absentee absorbed in doing other things.

Q: How can we help demented people feel more comfortable?

A: Use physical contact as your constant message that everything is all right and that you love the person you care for. It is rare that people find such touch unwelcome but, if they indicate this, respect it. For most people, touch is a message that gets through when words do not.

Lay your hand on the person's arm when you talk, gently rub his back or massage his shoulders, give her a hand massage. Any such physical movement should be slow, firm, and leisurely. Quick pats and tugs are very disturbing and unpleasant. If a hug is appropriate and welcome, a side-by-side hug is less threatening than a full frontal body hug, which can be very invasive. Do not use hugging as a way of patronizing people; they will detect your insincerity.

Q: I look after an old man with Alzheimer's who's always cursing at me. How can I make him stop?

A: The chances of changing him are slight. Either he has a lifelong habit of such behavior or it is part of his dementia. But you will probably feel better if you could set limits. It is important to be able to do so, even if the person cannot remember them.

It is appropriate to tell someone who is being verbally abusive, "I'm sorry you feel like that but I don't care to be spoken to this way." Such words do not necessarily stop the person with Alzheimer's, but they will make you as the caregiver feel less powerless.

Setting limits is not the same as trying to retrain someone.

Forget about that entirely. Trying to retrain someone with Alzheimer's is one of the biggest mistakes that caregivers find hard to let go of.

It is not easy to keep good communication going in Alzheimer's. However, if we listen with the heart, we will often comprehend what is really going on. Even when the words might fail to connect, we can still act with loving-kindness, knowing that kindness is always appropriate. This communicates the most necessary message of all: that our caring can be counted on. When the person with Alzheimer's understands that we care, the actual form of our communication is less important. Even the roadblocks and the cul-de-sacs do not matter anymore. The real and important message is love.

Dealing with Difficult Problems

This chapter is intended to help you look for solutions and ways of coping with day-to-day problems. The solutions may be obvious or they may require some innovative thinking or adjustment on your behalf. Not all problems necessarily have a solution. Sometimes the answer will be to try to change yourself.

Over the years, I have formulated a three-point plan to approach all problem solving. This plan helps both family members and professional care staff in their search for solutions to difficulties involving the care and needs of people with dementia. You too might find it useful to keep this in mind.

Ask yourself the following:
1. What is the feeling underlying this behavior?
2. What is the unmet need underlying this behavior?
3. How shall I meet this need?

There is only one major thing to remember: *All Alzheimer behaviors have meaning.*

Be sure you are honest about who has the problem. Many problem behaviors are only a problem to the caregiver. For example, if the problem is that someone is undressing in front of a window, you could close the curtains rather than fight about getting dressed again. This may not be the solution you wanted, but it may be the best workable solution for the situation.

The problems this chapter attempts to address are arranged alphabetically.

Abuse

Q: I help someone look after her mother. Last week when I got there, her mother was crying. She told me her daughter had been screaming at her because she put on a coffeepot without water in it. She seems afraid of her daughter. What should I do?

A: Verbal abuse qualifies as abuse as much as hitting someone. If you suspect the daughter is abusing her mother regularly and that this was not an isolated incident, you have a legal duty to report the daughter to the local senior services agency. Any such reporting will be in confidence.

Alzheimer's Association statistics report that up to 4 percent of the elderly are being abused. If 4 million Americans have Alzheimer's disease, that means some 160,000 elders with Alzheimer's are being abused.

Unfortunately, abuse and Alzheimer's disease go together. Because it is so stressful to cope with, often caregivers feel overwhelmed by too many demands made on their time and their energy. This can bring out the kinds of feelings that lead to abuse. Abuse can occur in a number of ways—physical, emotional, sexual, financial, as well as abuse through neglect and illegal restraint.

Such problems are seldom a result of mere cruelty. Usually a combination of factors causes people to injure those who need their help and protection. Overwhelming situations combined with personal inadequacies spill out in rage.

Q: I'm doing my best to look after my father with Alzheimer's, but I've got a husband who's sick, a son with a drug problem, and a daughter with an eating disorder. Sometimes I've hit my father. No one knows I do this and I'm so ashamed. I probably should never have had him live with us, but I promised my mother before she died. What can I do?

A: You need help from your local senior services, both for yourself and to find somewhere safe for your father to live. You're under so much stress right now that taking care of someone with dementia is overwhelming. You probably meant well in your promise to your mother, but even she would not have the right to expect you to take a person with dementia into an already overstretched household.

No one owes another person care for Alzheimer's. No one person can cope with another's dementia, and taking your father into your home can't work under these circumstances. You can't possibly give him what he needs by yourself. No one could.

Under stress, it's natural to feel angry at someone you are always looking after, but it is entirely wrong to hit, push, or physically punish that person. It is normal to feel like yelling sometimes, but you have to find ways to express those impulses without being abusive to the person in your charge. As soon as you feel that anger welling up, give yourself time out in a different room and stay there until you've taken ten deep breaths. Seek help.

Q: I think my sister is taking my mother's money out of her bank account and spending it on drugs. My mother has Alzheimer's so she can't do anything. Can I?

A: Yes, you can. Financial abuse of elders is as illegal as every other kind of abuse. In Alzheimer's, it is not unusual for financial abuse to occur, with a family member or sometimes even an outside caregiver taking financial advantage of the incompetent person. This must be reported by anyone who suspects it, and action can be taken by the justice system and by the social services system to safeguard the assets of an incompetent person.

Contact the local senior services or Agency on Aging to let them know of your concerns. They will investigate and can keep your complaint confidential.

Q: My wife, who has Alzheimer's, tells the neighbors I beat her up all the time. I don't. I really don't. How can I stop her from doing this?

A: You would do better to talk to the neighbors yourself and explain that your wife has Alzheimer's and that it is her dementia that makes her say untrue things about you.

Make sure you don't ever handle her so that there are bruises or other marks on her body, since it's possible that well-meaning neighbors could report you for suspected abuse.

It is rare that a demented person can accurately identify being abused. It is fairly common, however, for someone to claim that he or she is being abused when it is not true.

People can accuse others of stealing from them, of not feeding them, of hitting them or beating them when it is entirely untrue. This obviously complicates the issues.

Concerned people should keep an eye open for physical evidence that may suggest abuse—bruising, unexplained falls, broken bones—while also staying aware of the fact that all of these can result from legitimate accidents.

Sam and his wife, Mary, took care of Sam's mother, who had Alzheimer's. After they took her for an Alzheimer workup, they found themselves reported to the local senior services division for abuse when bruise marks were seen on her arm. They had never abused her. She was prone to easy bruising, as many older people are, and had probably acquired the marks when being helped up from a low armchair. The accusations shattered the couple. Soon after that they placed Sam's mother in a care home.

This sad story highlights the complexity of the abuse issue. We cannot emphasize the dangers enough, yet we must always beware of witch-hunts that label innocent caregivers as abusers.

Agitation

Q: Every night my aunt works herself up into a tantrum, about nothing most of the time. The rest of the time she's fine and mellow. What's happening?

A: She's sundowning—so-called because it refers to a period of agitation that typically occurs around sundown.

Many people with Alzheimer's have periods of agitation when they become anxious, worried, obsessive, fearful, or angry. It is common for this to occur in the late afternoon, typically between 3 P.M. and 7 P.M. This phenomenon is not peculiar to Alzheimer's disease. It is associated with many dementias and can also happen to older people who otherwise seem to be in good health.

There have been many suggestions as to why this occurs. It may well be much more widespread than we think, since mothers of young children often have similar problems with their fractious youngsters during this same time of day. People suffering a loss or depression report feeling worse at this time of day, so theorists guess that the agitation might be caused by a biochemical response to the fading of daylight.

What really matters is not the specific cause—since that cannot be clearly established at this point—but what you do about it. There are a number of ways to help alleviate this periodic agitation.

When someone shows agitation, we can reasonably guess that fear and insecurity are the two prime feelings being expressed. Create a sense of safety, be loving, and be prepared to divert your aunt at these difficult times.

Likely factors in agitation are:
• tiredness
• hunger
• boredom
• emotional distress caused by the day's events
• loneliness
• grief from the losses of old age
• fear caused by awareness that all is not well within
• feelings of being useless and unwanted

Many people, old and young alike, suffer an energy drop in the late afternoon. Since people with Alzheimer's often need constant activities to occupy them, it is easy to forget that they may also be exhausted by them. When sundowning is a regular event, try several of the following:

- Add an after-lunch nap to the routine. This can be a welcome opportunity for the caregiver to rest too, even perhaps curling up in the same bed or on the same comfortable sofa.
- If this is not acceptable, try extending morning sleeping hours by encouraging your aunt to stay in bed longer.
- Offer a snack in midafternoon to help avoid this energy drop—fruit and yogurt, fruit juice, or cake and coffee, for example.
- Play a beloved piece of music and sit with your arm around your aunt while listening or doing something else that works to calm her.
- Distract her from agitation by entertainment. Some people enjoy particular videos and will happily watch the same one day after day. Others enjoy comedy or discussion programs on television.
- Take a walk together, or go for a drive to someplace where you can sit and enjoy the view.
- Try using lavender essential oil diffused or sprayed in the room to help bring about emotional calmness. This really works.

Remember that agitation can be catching and do not allow yourself to be infected by it. Stay calm within, it will pass.

Q: My husband gets agitated every night before dinner. He often says he's worthless and even cries sometimes. I try to cheer him up but it's very hard. Is there any way I can stop these episodes?

A: What your husband says at this time is unlikely to be the actual cause of his agitation. His agitation comes from the multiple causes that underlie sundowning. What he says, even though it may have validity, is only the product of agitation.

That doesn't mean there's no truth in what he's saying. This is often when people refer to the themes that obsess them, commonly about one of their primary relationships—their parents, their spouse, or some other major figure in their life. Often they are expressing a sense of loss, anger, or anxiety.

Your husband's theme is his sense of lacking inner worth. This may well be a genuine sorrow, but it is only a part of his life. It passes as the agitation time is over. Many caregivers more or less ignore these themes—"Oh, she's just playing that same old tape again!"—but they are actually a crucial part of an individual's resolution.

Wise caregivers find ways to help the sick person resolve the issues if possible, since they contribute to the underlying anxieties that trouble the patient.

It may be helpful to listen responsively and offer emotional support. This is the way that growth and resolution are made possible, even with the memory failure and cognitive limitations typical of Alzheimer's.

The resolution comes with the acceptance of unconditional love, and this is certainly the basic relationship of caregiving. The life of the heart does not cease just because the brain is afflicted.

Alcohol

Q: My parents always drank a lot. Now my mom has Alzheimer's and they still drink as much. Is this okay?

A: It may not be okay. Some of the problems of Alzheimer's may be exaggerated through overuse of alcohol. It is also true that the alcoholic is likely to prove to be a more difficult type of Alzheimer's patient.

Early Alzheimer symptoms can be masked by or mistaken for alcoholism, especially if the person is self-medicating emotional pain by drinking. When actress Rita Hayworth was beginning to manifest Alzheimer's disease, people assumed that she was an alcoholic. Once the disease has been diagnosed, unfortunately, the patterns of destructive behavior associated with heavy alcohol use are likely to remain. In fact, difficult personality traits are merely increased by the progress of Alzheimer's disease.

In cases of mild drinking, there may be no reason a person should not continue. In the case of a couple who have always indulged in heavy drinking together, there is the question of whether continuing this is actually an abuse of the partner with Alzheimer's.

Anger

Q: I'm tired of looking after my husband. He's got dementia and he's driving me crazy too. I want to keep him home, but I get so angry it scares me. What can I do to help myself and him?

A: First, take an honest look at your anger issues around being a caregiver. If you have continuous responsibility for a person with Alzheimer's, you probably get very tired, lonely, and fed-up from time to time. Under such circumstances small irritations can lead to feeling a great deal of anger.

Since it's your husband who has Alzheimer's, you may have feelings of anger that are really connected with your sense of loss. Perhaps you feel that his illness has stolen what was once yours, as well as stealing away your future dreams of having a good retirement together. It's natural to feel angry toward a partner who can no longer fulfill the balancing role you once appreciated.

I hope you are already attending a regular support group and that you will also consider going into therapy so that you can explore your deepest feelings and learn how to cope. Also, please add a stress management class and a care plan for yourself that includes exercise (a great stress reducer) as well as making sure you follow a good diet.

Q: My mother and I used to be very close. We were more like best friends than mother and daughter. Now she's so affected by Alzheimer's disease, I find I can't bear to be near her. It sounds horrible, I know, but

I feel so angry with her. I know it's not her fault, but how can I stop my own feelings?

A: You can't stop your feelings without understanding their source. Intense anger can often underlie changes in a relationship. If, for example, you now have to take care of your mother as if she were your child, this can be shocking. If you once admired your mother and she now behaves in ways that frighten or disgust you, you may well feel angry.

Only you know exactly why you feel angry. You could usefully give some thought to this: Is it because you're afraid of Alzheimer's? Do you secretly think your mother could choose to manage better? Is it because you feel overworked, unappreciated, and lonely, now that you no longer have your original relationship with your mother? Do you feel like an orphan? Do you get enough sleep? Are you grieving? How does her condition hurt you? Anger usually covers something that wounds you, so ask yourself what hurts.

Accepting the necessary change of role can be very hard and asks a great deal of you. However, accepting such a change at least gives you a chance to have some relationship, as opposed to none, and you may find consolation in this acceptance.

Most caregivers feel angry occasionally. Some feel angry often or even all the time. It is not wrong necessarily. Unfortunately, anger reduces your ability to be a good caregiver. It is also hard work. It uses up energy you need for other things, like enjoying life. It reduces your ability to feel compassion. As you know, it makes you feel guilty too and takes away your sense of humor altogether. Therefore, you need to help yourself if you often feel angry.

One way to start helping yourself is to become very clear about what exactly is making you feel angry. Make a list of all the reasons. This will help you see what is involved, since there are often multiple factors behind anger.

Please consider both counseling and a support group to help you cope with this situation.

Q: My husband gets furious very easily now that he has Alzheimer's. How can I control this, and will it get worse?

A: It sounds as if your husband has been recently diagnosed, which probably means he is in a fairly early stage of the disease. This is typically when anger is most likely to arise. Your husband is undoubtedly becoming aware of his losses and becoming very frightened.

You and the rest of his family can help him by being prepared to talk about the reality of his situation. All too often, family members decide not to mention the illness, thus condemning the sick person to terrible loneliness.

The most important thing to understand is that all anger is based on something that is real to the person with Alzheimer's. It is not a disease symptom but a reaction to something going on. Your task will be to figure out what your husband is reacting to in each situation. Look for something that he might feel is threatening him, since this is the usual pattern in outbreaks of anger.

Sometimes, sadly, the anger that has been stifled over the years begins to emerge because the person is losing his or her inhibitions. These are the people you sometimes hear about, the mild-mannered man who becomes a raging tyrant. Alzheimer's experts report that these people were often angry before but kept the anger within. Such rages, however, are not the typical rages of Alzheimer's, which tend to be fierce and short.

Dealing with these outbursts, it is best to begin by acknowledging the anger: "I know it must be so frustrating when you can't find the words." Comments like this can help by showing that you understand. Sometimes, it might be best to let the anger express itself. You can make appropriate comments in a calm, soothing voice. That shows you care and that you can accept the anger.

When your husband gets mad, step back and give him some space, instead of moving forward to intervene. Remember that anger says, "back off!" It is unlikely he will pursue you to hit you, so just step out of range. Other ways to deal with rages include distraction. Initiate a new activity, take the person into another room or out of the house, or go for a drive. (Being in a car feels safe and cozy, and the change of scenery is pleasantly entertaining without being demanding.)

Another approach is to ignore the anger. This can be done either by remaining with your husband or by leaving the room while he expresses his anger. If you do this—and it can be useful for him to have the literal space in which to spill out emotions—make it clear why you are leaving and that your absence is not punitive.

Alzheimer anger can be very invasive, since the person often blames the caregiver. Try not to take the outburst personally, even if personal remarks are made. It makes sense that anyone suffering the great losses and limitations of the disease would feel angry.

Behavior Problems

Q: When I take my wife out, she sometimes does things that other people find very peculiar. For example, she spits. I don't know why, but she seems to have excess saliva since she got Alzheimer's. Should I explain to people that she's sick?

A: Absolutely yes, you should explain to people. Usually, they are very kind about such lapses once they understand what's going on. The saliva problem is unusual, but one family dealt with it by giving their mother chewing gum, and this seemed to control her need to spit.

Try never to feel embarrassed by your wife's behavior, since she may pick up your agitation and reflect it back to you. Remember that her illness has removed both her normal judgment and inhibitions. The results may include a wide range of odd behaviors, from spitting to taking out false teeth in public and washing them in a coffee cup.

Nearly all our social behavior is learned and therefore can be unlearned in the course of a brain-impairing disease. The best way to cope with odd behavior in someone with Alzheimer's is to show the same humor, understanding, and kindness you would with a child. Indicate what you would like the person to do in a nonjudgmental manner. "It probably isn't such a good idea to wash your teeth in your coffee. Maybe you could pop them back into your mouth right now."

This kind of leading suggestion usually works well, especially if you keep criticism out of your tone.

Catastrophic Reaction

Q: I took my grandmother, who has dementia, out for a walk last week. We were walking across the grass when the sprinklers went on. Well, you should have heard her yell! I thought she was going to have a heart attack. What was going on?

A: Your grandmother was having a catastrophic reaction. This means overreaction to an event or stimulus, either in the form of anger, fear, anxiety, grief, or some other emotionally powerful way.

This reaction probably happened because your grandmother no longer cognitively knows that water will come rushing out of a sprinkler and the sudden event frightened her. She did not understand what was going on, why the water was pouring out, or what she should do about it.

In other situations, overreaction may arise because the person with Alzheimer's misinterprets a situation.

Q: My wife was watching TV the other day. Suddenly she started screaming, "I haven't stolen anything. I'm not a thief!" I had to calm her down. Was this some kind of hallucination?

A: Possibly, but it's more likely that something in the television program set her off. Sometimes it's hard for people with dementia to understand that television isn't real, or that what they see on it is contained inside the screen.

For example, seeing a fire shown on television, someone with dementia may want to call 911. There are many ways a person with dementia can misunderstand and misinterpret everything. Such mistakes are common and are probably not hallucinations in the usual sense.

If your wife had dozed off for a moment, perhaps she had a dream that set her off. She may have had a memory that stirred her up. If this happens, soothe and comfort her and then, when appropriate, distract her with some other activity.

Other catastrophic reactions may be brought about by caregivers intervening too roughly or too quickly. Never confront; always persuade. Never give orders; make suggestions. Never push or pull roughly; always guide gently. Show violence and you will receive violence. When you try to force someone with Alzheimer's to do something, you are treating that person as an object, not as a human being, and you are likely to be taught an unpleasant lesson in return.

Most catastrophic reactions are soon over and forgotten. Although they are emotionally powerful at the time, they are really insignificant.

Confrontation

Q: We're three sisters trying to help our mother, who has just been diagnosed with Alzheimer's. We're still trying to get her to admit she has Alzheimer's. How can we make her admit this?

A: You can't. Don't waste time trying to confront your mother. Confrontation never works with people with Alzheimer's disease. You will only bring about a catastrophic reaction.

If you are trying to prove your mother wrong through rational explanation, she will react badly because she has an impaired ability to follow rational thought.

I wonder why you are so determined that she should accept her illness. Are you trying to get her to acknowledge weakness, or trying to force change on her she isn't ready for? She may well need more care than she's prepared to admit, in which case you will get better results simply if you put in place the kind of help she needs and do it tactfully and kindly. She doesn't have to acknowledge her needs for help.

What her resistance tells you is that she needs the protection of her denial right now. The more gentle you and your sisters are about getting her needs met, the more she can risk trusting you. Only when she feels safe will she let go of her denial.

Remember, you will never win an argument with someone who has dementia.

If you are being confrontational, ask yourself why. Chances are you are feeling angry and not really admitting it. You'll find it helps to deal with your own anger without trying to make your mother wrong. She will always be wrong from now on, because she has Alzheimer's disease and that's what it does to mental functioning.

Dehydration

Q: My mother has Alzheimer's but she also has other health problems, and a visiting nurse comes to see her several times a week. The nurse says we need to get Mother to drink plenty of water. Why do we have to do this? How can we persuade Mother to do it, since she doesn't like drinking water?

A: Everyone needs to drink plenty of water daily, up to six eight-ounce glasses or more. Lack of sufficient water increases dementia and confusion symptoms and is a main cause for constipation, which also increases dementia and confusion.

Dehydration is so frequent a problem among older people that it merits special attention. Some experts think the thirst mechanism becomes deficient in old age, while others consider that the effects of medications may somehow dismantle the body's natural thirst defenses.

Whatever the cause, dehydration is common. People simply do not drink enough water and do not feel thirsty. Additionally, many older people, probably like your mother, were never in the habit of drinking enough water and often dislike it.

Tea, coffee, milk, alcohol, and soft drinks do not count toward the water quota. Add a touch of fruit juice or squeeze some lemon into the water to give it some flavor. Offer many small drinks a day rather than a few large ones. Try an herbal tea without caffeine.

Tell your mother her doctor says she must drink water. This often works for those who respect their doctor as an authority figure. Don't make a fight of it, however. It's not worth it.

Driving

Q: My dad may have Alzheimer's. We can't get him to the doctor, and meanwhile we're all scared to death about him driving. Should we stop him? If so, how? I know he won't want to give up his independence.

A: Undoubtedly he shouldn't be driving. No one with dementia should be driving. Most states require doctors to report patients with dementia so their licenses can be pulled.

Of course, everyone knows how important it is to be free to drive. It is often the biggest factor in keeping a sense of independence in an older person like your father. In a way, to lose his car is to lose his ability to manage life.

However, recent research reveals that about 40 percent of people diagnosed with dementia had a road accident or caused one in the six months before diagnosis. Think how you'd feel if your father caused someone's death with his bad driving. And, if someone with Alzheimer's has any trauma, such as a car accident, it invariably brings about a decline in general ability to manage and a further step down in the course of the disease. Therefore, it is not the kindness it may seem to be to let your father continue driving until the inevitable accident.

Get his doctor's help in stopping him from driving. Be sure to put an alternative transportation plan into effect immediately so he can still get around.

Eating

Q: My mother's eating has changed since she got dementia. For example, she won't eat different foods if they touch each other on her plate. Then she eats everything on one side of the plate, then everything on the other. Why?

A: I don't think anyone knows exactly what causes these anomalies in Alzheimer's—possibly brain damage or changes in perception—but they are quite common.

Problems with eating can take a number of forms: eating too much, too little, too slowly, or too often. The answer comes usually in the caregiver quietly taking necessary action, not in trying to convince the person with dementia to change.

Q: My wife eats whole boxes of Eskimo Pies. She just goes to the re-frigerator and takes them until they're gone. The doctor says she's got to lose some weight. How can I control her eating?

A: Don't buy them and she can't eat them. She is very unlikely to go out and buy her own. If she asks you to, say "We'll see," just as all good parents learn to do.

Most people with Alzheimer's develop an intense hunger for sugar, in the form of ice cream, cake, cookies, or candy. Sugar imbalance may be part of this. It may also be caused by overdrive in the system that demands constant caloric input, with sugar being the most popular item desired.

Q: My doctor wants me to put my husband on a low cholesterol diet. Bill loves to eat. Why shouldn't he enjoy his food?

A: I'm with you on this one. We need to ask ourselves what we are saving people for—so they can "do" good Alzheimer's disease? You may simply consider it not worth the struggle. In my non-medical opinion, as long as a person with Alzheimer's is not grossly overweight or diabetic, rigid diets are not as important as they once might have been. Putting a person who already has a terminal and profoundly limiting illness on a healthier diet seems irrelevant.

Q: When I ask my mother what she wants to eat, she always says she's not hungry. Should I wait for her to feel hungry?

A: No, go ahead, cook the food and serve it. You don't mention that she doesn't actually eat, so I'm assuming she does eat what you set in front of her.

Some people get hungrier with dementia, others become indifferent to food. Typically people gain weight as they grow more ill, exercise less, and indulge their whims, then lose weight as the illness progresses. You must decide for yourself what your values are on this issue.

A number of people lose interest in food but will eat when it is set before them. We know that people with dementia usually lose their sense of smell. This means that food becomes tasteless to them. You might want to spice food up accordingly.

Q: My mother-in-law always says, "I don't want to eat. I'm not hungry," and I have to fight with her over every meal. Help!

A: It sounds as if food has become the battleground between you and that maybe you could learn from good mothers who deal with their children's power struggles over food.

Since I seriously doubt that your mother-in-law would let herself starve to death, why not just place the food in front of her and leave it? If she says she's not hungry, just airily say, "Oh well, I'll just leave it there right now, that's okay." I suspect she will go ahead and eat. Leave the food as long as necessary. Don't let eating be a battleground.

Q: My father is very disabled now. The doctor says he's in the terminal stage of Alzheimer's. He can't really seem to chew and is losing weight, but we don't want to put him in a nursing home. How can we make him eat?

A: Try making high-protein shakes for your father. They will supply everything he needs nutritionally. A shake does not have

CHAPTER 7

to include milk. You could use soy milk, fruit juice, ice cream, yogurt, nondairy creamers, and add fruits, eggs, vitamin supplements, wheat germ, and protein powder.

If your father is approaching the end of his life, you need to begin to think about your choices in this regard—for example, whether he wishes to have life support through artificial feeding or other interventions.

Forgetfulness

Q: Everyone says how forgetting things is the sign of Alzheimer's, but surely we all forget things, don't we?

A: The forgetfulness of Alzheimer's is a profound forgetting, allied with global loss of abilities to think, reason, cope with life routines, and structure daily existence.

Until we know someone who has severe memory problems, most of us cannot imagine how deeply it cuts through the fabric of life. Our lives as human beings depend on the fact that our mind weaves together our past and our present to make our future. Once we cannot rely on our minds to perform the weaving function, daily life unravels.

In Alzheimer's disease, short-term memory goes first, sometimes followed by fracturing of long-term memory, although most people retain some parts of long-term memory to a surprising degree. Effectively, this means that at first the main problems are ones of forgetfulness in daily life, similar to those experienced by most people. Typically, the difference is that people with Alzheimer's may have less awareness of their forgetting.

Things will not come back to them later, as happens to normal people. Eventually, they forget entire days. In this early stage, there is also an accompanying loss of cognitive ability, which is experienced by family members as a vague sense of something being not quite right, although they can't put their finger on it.

The pattern of forgetfulness varies, probably according to the person's former mind habits, and this variation often deceives

120

people at first into thinking that the person with Alzheimer's could remember things if he or she chose to do so. Many people who retain excellent long-term memory can tell every detail of their childhood but do not know who was sitting with them five minutes ago.

Q: Would it be a good idea to label things in the house so our grandmother knows what's in which closet and so on? Should we have a daily bulletin board so she knows our routine?

A: Try each idea and see what happens. Written notes can be useful reminders and they help to keep some people functional for quite a long time. It can also be useful to label drawers and cupboards as reminders of where certain necessary things can be found, if that is meaningful for the individual.

You will soon see if this works for your grandmother. Some people can't comprehend written information or it may not even register in their minds. If this is your grandmother's case, these efforts won't help her. The most important thing is to realize that the decline in memory cannot really be held back by such reminders.

Sometimes, entire houses are labeled from top to bottom by well-meaning caregivers in an effort to help the person with Alzheimer's. In fact, overdoing this is merely confusing. However, labeling items that represent the most important daily needs of the person with Alzheimer's may be helpful. For example, good use of labeling in the kitchen may include: "Cheerios," "milk," and "cat food."

Q: Sometimes my father seems to think the present is the past. Should I keep reminding him what year this is?

A: When memory goes, the person may forget what year it is. The ship of memory can anchor anywhere without the person knowing the difference. If someone is living in the memory year of 1932, this is not craziness. It is the logical result of memory loss.

You will find your father sets his own limits on this. Either he will accept what you say or he will more or less ignore it because it won't make sense to him. Don't struggle to convince him. Just let it go. It doesn't really matter all that much what day or even what year this is in his life. What matters is how safe, how happy, and how loved he feels.

Hoarding

Q: My mother lives in a nursing home now and the nurses tell me they keep finding food in her night-table drawer. Why is she collecting food? Do you think they aren't feeding her enough?

A: I'm sure they're feeding her enough, even though it might not be very interesting food.

Your mother is hoarding food because it represents some form of security for her at a deep emotional level. Hoarding of various things is not uncommon in Alzheimer's and is an emotional barometer. There would be no point in trying to train your mother not to do this, nor in reproaching her.

There are many forms of hoarding. Betty has twenty-two cans of blackberries in her cupboard, which she bought because she liked the picture on the label. Mabel has fifty-three Kleenexes in her handbag. George hides money. So far, several hundred dollars have gone missing but no one knows where he has hidden them. Maria, who lives in a care home, has sixteen stuffed animals jammed into her bedside locker; she collected them from other residents' rooms.

Several varieties of hoarding seem to be common to people with Alzheimer's. The most difficult is the hoarding or hiding of money. The money is effectively lost until it can be rediscovered by the caregiver. The afflicted person may accuse others of stealing.

Such false accusations have sometimes been classified medically as evidence of paranoia. It is not evidence of paranoia, however, but the logical result of hiding things and having no memory of having done so. Naturally, under such conditions, it looks to the person with Alzheimer's as if someone else has taken the money.

Hoarding is a natural response to fear and insecurity. It is the way in which the person with Alzheimer's is trying to keep the universe under control, particularly in the areas that especially worry the individual. Some worry about money most, and they will hide it from potential thieves. Others worry about food, so they hide that. Still others collect particular things that presumably represent security or pleasure to them.

No one likes to be without money. It represents independence and power. Therefore, a workable solution needs to be found that will allow the person to have some money without losing large sums. You might discuss the issue and find an acceptable sum that makes the person feel secure. One woman was content with a five-dollar bill being left in her purse for her daily. Another woman received $300 twice a month. Another man had a pile of play money and did not know the difference. The answer depends on how much the person needs and knows.

Q: I get so mad because other residents at my mother's care home are always taking her things. Is there some way to stop them?

A: Does this worry your mother or does it worry only you? If it's you, perhaps you can come to terms with it.

People with dementias often have no sense of possession. They may claim other people's things as their own and guard them fiercely, while showing no wish to safeguard what is really theirs.

It is a problem, but, as with so many other Alzheimer problems, it's understandable. These people have forgotten what is theirs. They may feel other people's things look like theirs, or they may just want to have them and therefore believe they own them.

There is no point in scolding someone with Alzheimer's for taking things or hoarding or hiding them. It is a memory problem, not a moral problem. It is cruel and meaningless to berate the person for things that cannot be helped. I know you care, but I suspect your mother doesn't.

Hygiene

Q: *We can't get my grandfather to take showers anymore and he's starting to smell of urine. How can we make him bathe more often?*

A: Hygiene becomes a problem for a number of people with Alzheimer's, although it is usually troubling to the caregiver rather than to the afflicted person, who is no longer aware of old, well-established habits of cleanliness.

Remember that the sloppiness or downright self-neglect that sometimes develops is only a disease process. To be clean according to the standards of society is not instinctive knowledge. It is a product of childhood training. Therefore, in dementia it is forgotten.

Your grandfather probably is not aware of his condition. He needs help, either to remind him to bathe or to physically assist him. If you can't do that, consider bringing in a bathing aide.

To keep this from being stressful, don't make a big deal of any of it. Treat the maintenance of cleanliness and hygiene as simply another task with which your grandfather needs help. Do not nag or scold because memory loss has removed his former standards. Just deal with it.

Smelling of urine is not so much a product of not bathing as it is of some physical loss of control. Either he may be losing physical control of his bladder, or perhaps he's forgetting to go to the bathroom until it's too late. Consider whether he needs someone to live with him full-time. He may need cueing to go to the bathroom.

It is especially important not to scold when incontinence or bowel control is the issue. See the section on incontinence for a fuller explanation.

Q: Since my mother's had Alzheimer's, she seems very reluctant to get in the shower. Why is this?

A: Many people with dementia seem to become afraid of showering. We don't know for sure why, but we can make some guesses. Perhaps the whole business of bathing may seem too overwhelmingly complex to the person with Alzheimer's, who may have forgotten how to do the hygiene routine properly. Perhaps it is puzzling.

Perhaps these people have forgotten that when they stand under a shower, at some point water will rush out on their heads. There they are, standing peacefully minding their own business, when—whoosh!—out comes a violent stream of water. The event is shocking and possibly unpleasantly stimulating.

Instead of a shower, try running a warm bath, maybe adding soap bubbles to make it appealing. This works well for a lot of people. Or, try getting your mother to sit in the shower on a shower stool and use a hand-held shower, avoiding getting water on her face. Use the shower head in gentle upward movements, starting from her feet, talking reassuringly all the time.

If this fails, you might try soaking a towel in hot water and wrapping it around her body. This feels good and might lead to more feelings of trust developing, which would allow you to continue the washing process.

If you are going to wash her hair, avoid running water straight onto her head. Instead, place your own hand on her hair and let the water run on your hand first. This avoids any shock or unpleasant physical feelings about the process.

It is really not worth your while to create a battle over this any more than you have to. Remember that many older people grew up in times when a bath once a week was considered respectable, with a wash and wipe sufficing for everyday cleansing. A good bath or shower once a week really is sufficient for cleanliness provided you can get some daily cooperation on washing. At a very basic level, people should wash under their arms and in and around the genitals.

Various people report success with a number of approaches to personal hygiene. For example, you could get a big container of baby wipes and persuade your charge to use them for self-cleansing after going to the toilet. People who hate to have their hair washed might allow it in the context of a hairdresser's shop.

If all else fails, you could try a respite center that includes showers and bathing as part of its routine. Strangers might get more cooperation than you do.

Q: This is embarrassing for me, but my mother won't clean herself after going to the bathroom. How do we get her to do this?

A: Try not to feel embarrassed. She's impaired by her illness, that's all. And you may be affected by the weird attitudes we have in general in this country around bodily functions.

Many people with Alzheimer's simply forget to clean themselves appropriately after using the bathroom. Be sure to have the toilet paper where it is visible and easily accessible. Even so, you may still have to give reminders and perhaps hand out toilet paper. You may even have to be prepared to wipe her yourself if need be. If so, take a good handful of paper and wipe from front to back, never from the anus forward.

If you are going to regularly clean up your mother after she uses the toilet, you should buy thin surgical gloves to keep your hands clean. They come in big packs like tissue handkerchief packs. While you may feel this to be humiliating for your mother, the chances are that she will not. Someone who has gone far enough along in her or his illness to forget the process has probably also lost the inhibition that made it shameful. In fact, it is no more shameful than needing help with dressing or shopping. It is we who feel it shameful because of the often peculiar attitudes our society has toward elimination and defecation.

Q: My husband wants to sleep in the same clothing he wears in the daytime. How can I stop him?

A: You must not have enough to worry about! Let him. It's not serious in the big picture of your caring for him.

If the real problem is that his clothes need washing, you will have to be cunning and wait your opportunity to snatch the clothes away.

Some people can only get hold of dirty clothing on the rare occasions when they can get their charge into the shower. Others do it by saying the person has to get changed for a special occasion or for a visit to the doctor.

Incontinence

Q: *My mother doesn't remember to go to the bathroom and has become incontinent. There's a good care home near here but they won't take her while she's incontinent. Is there a way to train her?*

A: No, but I doubt that your mother is genuinely incontinent. Incontinence is used as a general term to mean loss of bowel or bladder control, but it is often used incorrectly. Someone who has forgotten to go to the bathroom because of memory loss is not strictly incontinent. Neither is it incontinence if a person does not know where the bathroom is anymore or cannot recognize the correct container for toilet purposes and therefore urinates in a waste basket. If a person has become so impaired that he or she cannot recognize the symptoms of needing to urinate or defecate, that is not strictly incontinence; it is dementia.

You may think it does not matter, since the results may be the same. However, the important difference is that someone who is impaired by Alzheimer's does not necessarily become incontinent. Even in nursing homes, as much as 90 percent of residents with Alzheimer's need not be incontinent during the daytime as long as staff take them regularly to the bathroom.

Home caregivers need to know the heartening news that as many as 90 percent of those with Alzheimer's can remain continent with helpful reminders. A two-hour schedule is adequate for most people. Additionally, always ensure a bathroom visit is made before leaving home and after getting back. Don't ask if your mother wants to go to the bathroom, since this may often evoke the answer, "No, I don't need to." Instead, suggest it in a positive way. "Okay, why don't we just make a bathroom call before we go out?" Keep it low-key. Should you start to make it a major issue, you may create the stress that leads to loss of control.

Make sure your mother doesn't have a bladder infection causing incontinence problems, and check that none of her medications could be causing this.

Paranoia

Q: Our uncle says the neighbors are breaking into the house at night and stealing things. (They aren't.) The doctor says he's got paranoia. Is this a different problem from Alzheimer's or are they connected?

A: Paranoia is often cited as being one of the problem symptoms of Alzheimer's disease. However, usually what might look like paranoia is a rational response to living inside the fractured mental abilities brought about by the disease. In other words, it is usually not paranoia but a reasonable fear response, given the limitations of the disease.

We often are unimaginative about this. The memory problems of Alzheimer's mean that people think their possessions have disappeared. Often, they misinterpret the world around them. Things are misheard or even mistranslated within the mind. Becoming fearful and insecure, their sense of safety is eroded.

It is personal memory that makes us feel safe. Because of our memory, we know our routine, we know who our friends are, we have a general plan and schedule that directs our lives. The person with Alzheimer's has none of these supports, and it is out of this that the often mentioned paranoia arises. It isn't paranoia—it is fear.

We need to be extremely sensitive to these issues within the lives of those with Alzheimer's. With that sensitivity, we can help create a new sense of security.

It is very likely that, if your uncle does not have someone living with him, this is the time to start planning for that so that he can feel supported and secure in his home.

Repetitive Questions

Q: My husband keeps asking the same question over and over again. He's driving me crazy. I know he can't remember what I tell him and that it's not his fault, but I need to make him stop. How?

A: Repetitive questions are one major reason why people seek help coping with Alzheimer's. Nothing can drive a caregiver more crazy than being asked the same question dozens, scores, or even hundreds of times a day.

You may think there is no solution. After all, the essence of this problem is that the person with Alzheimer's does not recall asking the question or receiving the answer. Repetitive questions are part of the disease process and many people ask them. The form of the question, however, is very significant. Everyone has an individual version of the question, and it is the nature of the question that gives the clue to its solution. The solution lies in answering the need beneath the question. Here are some examples.

"What time is it?" asks Lee, for the eighth time in an hour.

"When can I go home?" asks Hannah, sitting in her own home.

"Are my mother and father coming home now?" asks eighty-eight-year-old Annie.

When caregivers only answer the questions asked, the answer will have to be repeated endlessly. People ask repetitive questions in response to a feeling within which they cannot express, either because they do not recognize it or because they cannot verbalize it.

Lee asks what time it is because he is bored and anxious. All the things he used to do are outside his abilities now, and his wife never thinks of asking him to do what little he can. His question is really a statement about how it feels to be stranded in an endless present with nothing to do. His wife would find relief from hearing that irritating question if she would let him help her—

sweep a floor, wash vegetables, wipe a tabletop, do some weeding. He may do none of it very well, but she would get relief from his question and he would get relief from his consuming boredom.

Hannah asks when she can go home, even as she sits in her home, because she does not recognize anything around her. Home means familiarity, security, the comfort of routine and habit, of knowing one's place in the world. Because she has Alzheimer's, she will never be at home again in the cognitive sense. However, she can be helped to *feel* at home. "This is your home. You've lived here about ten years but you forget because you have an illness that makes you forget things," says her caregiver, putting an arm around Hannah.

Annie asks about her parents because they were her primary relationship. She never married, always lived at home, and, although she had a good professional job, she never became emotionally independent. When she feels insecure, she immediately asks about her parents.

Try not to let repetitive questions get to you. Anger will make compassion impossible and your relationship will deteriorate and may turn into blaming the person who is ill for the very symptoms of the illness. Once you uncover their real meanings, you will probably find more patience to bear the questions.

Safety

Q: I'm worried about my mother's safety in the house while I'm at work. Once I came home and found she'd put sheets in the oven and switched it on—to warm them up, she said. How can I make sure she's okay?

A: I'm glad you're looking into this, since safety is the biggest worry for many caregivers. It has many aspects, including your mother wandering away, fire hazards, dangerous appliances.

It is very important for your mother to be wearing identification. Never assume she would not walk out of the house and get lost. It only needs to happen once to be a disaster. Get a Medic-Alert bracelet and have it inscribed with her name and phone number and the legend "memory impaired." If she is ever found wandering and lost, the finder will call the national 1-800 number on the bracelet or your own phone number. Most people are familiar with the Medic-Alert system. Make sure you have a good, clear, recent picture of your mother, in case she ever gets lost.

Alert your neighbors, too. Ask them to let you know if your relative wanders out alone. Often an entire neighborhood becomes a friendly guardian system to help support a family.

Safety at home means childproofing the house for an adult who has had a lifetime of using all the things that suddenly you do not wish him or her to use. Do not waste your energy on trying to retrain your mother. Instead, put your energy into making your house safe. Turn all stove switches off, and remove the knobs themselves if necessary. Gas and electric stoves have one main energy control: use it. Switch the stove off at the main and do not ever forget to do this if you are going to leave the person alone in the house.

There is a fireproof hood system that will dump chemicals over a stove fire if pots burn, but this kind of thing does not come cheap. You may find it easier to get the kind of stove that has a lid that can be lowered to cover all burners. It is tedious to do all this, but it ensures safety.

Remove or immobilize all hazards. If your mother is no longer able, for example, to regulate the shower, turn down your water temperature so she can't scald herself. Never trust your mother to take medication in the right quantities. Measure out each dose and then put the medication away securely.

Consider enrolling your mother in a day activity program, since that would provide the safety and supervision she needs. Or at least have someone look in on her during the day.

Sexuality

Q: My mother wants to get married again, so she's always trying to have dates. She has dementia and I'm not sure what to do about this.

A: Having dementia doesn't mean no one will ever love her again, neither does it make her hopes inappropriate, necessarily. I have known ladies with dementia who have happily pursued affairs of the heart. It probably does mean that you might have to supervise the suitability of any prospective suitors, although you are not required to actively go out and solicit them for her!

Just be sure that the relationship is not abusive physically, sexually, or financially. Also, be sure her estate is safe from fortune hunters.

Q: My father has always been a very respectable man. Because of his increasing dementia, we had to put him in a nursing home. The nurses say he keeps touching their breasts and trying to fondle them. I'm shocked by this. Why would he do such terrible things?

A: The usual social inhibitions against such behavior are being eroded by his disease. His conduct is not the outrage it would be from a fully cognitive person. He really can't help it, and I'm sure the nurses can cope with him, even if they don't like to. Maybe you need to remind everyone that he is demented. Speak to the director of nursing if necessary.

Old men with dementia might sometimes become uninhibited, but they never become rapists. His actions may also represent his loneliness and need for contact, not really of a sexual nature. Perhaps if you could think of ways to help your father feel less isolated, less afraid, that might help him adjust to living in care, which is a very lonely situation for most people.

Of course, his actions may also be the expression of the fact that sexuality still lives as a vital force in him.

Q: My father has had to put my stepmother into a care home because she has really bad Alzheimer's. He brings her home on weekends sometimes and he indicated that they still have an active sex life. Don't you think that's disgusting?

A: No. People do not necessarily lose their sexuality nor their capacity to express it until the later stages of Alzheimer's. A married couple may still have a full sexual life together; and an unmarried person can still successfully undertake and continue love affairs.

Some adult children find this shocking and think that, for example, a man should not want to make love to his impaired wife. Sometimes adult children feel they should prevent an impaired parent from forming a sexual relationship with another adult.

This really comes out of our general feeling in this society that disabled people are not, or should not be, or should not even want to be, sexual beings—even more so if they are old and disabled. Even more again if they have adult children who can't respect their rights and private life.

How your father and stepmother work out their sexuality is no one's business but their own.

Q: *Since our mother is now in a nursing home, our father wants to start seeing a woman from the senior center. We think this is completely wrong. He says he's lonely. We try to see him when we can, but we have very busy lives. What do you think?*

A: I think you should respect your father's choices. The man is effectively a widower now. This is a complex matter that basically should be left to the adult concerned with it. Unfortunately, often the adult children expect the unimpaired spouse to sit alone night after night in an empty house that is no longer a home. Yet those same adult children give little of their time to the healthy parent. That is a heavy additional burden of loneliness for an already suffering human being to carry.

If you expect to have any influence at all, you should at least be working hard at including your father in your lives. Otherwise, mind your own business.

Sleep

Q: I'm desperate for sleep. Ever since my husband's had Alzheimer's, he doesn't seem to know day from night. He gets up in the night and expects me to do the same. Should we get sleeping pills for him?

A: Sleep problems in Alzheimer's are actually waking problems, the most frequent being nighttime wakefulness. Often the person with Alzheimer's loses all real sense of time even though he can still read the time on a clock. Time just does not mean anything cognitively anymore. So when he wakes up, he gets up.

Someone gets up in the night on impulse through lack of tiredness, because it feels like time to get up, to go to the bathroom, to explore, to get something to eat or drink—for all kinds of reasons. It scarcely matters what the reason is. What matters is what you do about it.

There is no reason why your husband cannot wander about the house at night as long as there is no danger in it. If you can't sleep when he does this, negotiate him back to bed if you can. Perhaps a gentle back rub will help, or a glass of hot milk and a cookie, or listening to a soothing tape.

The real problem is that you have to be able to sleep. No one can go long with interrupted nights, especially if there is stressful daytime work to be done.

If possible, get other helpers to sleep overnight so that you can sleep. If that is impossible, you may finally have to resort to sleeping medications, but be aware that this comes at great cost. There are few satisfactory major sleep medications for people with Alzheimer's. They all have unfortunate side effects, some of which can greatly increase the confusion, agitation, and impairment of the disease.

Try the following. A hospital in Leicester, England, has found that using lavender essential oil, diffused throughout a room at night, soothes and calms people with dementia so they are better able to sleep.

Following my recommendation, a dementia unit in Newport, Oregon, tried this and found behavior changes immediately in their residents—more calm, less agitation. You can buy these products at health stores, beauty stores, and alternative medicine stores.

Undressing

Q: My aunt keeps taking her clothes off in public. We want to know how to stop this.

A: Some people go through a stage of undressing in public, and this can be hard for caregivers to deal with. However, people with Alzheimer's have no sense that it is not appropriate. I'm sure your aunt doesn't even know or care that this bothers you. We can only guess why she's doing this—maybe it feels good to be naked, perhaps her clothes are uncomfortable, possibly she's simply expressing some kind of emotional vulnerability, or just needs something interesting to do.

It is a hard problem to deal with since the urge seems to be quite persistent while it is present. Nursing homes often deal with it either by tying people up or by drugging them into submission, both of which are extremely questionable in terms of medical ethics, forms of abuse that are now illegal in all states.

Some caregivers solve the problem by adapting. If they are inside the home, they draw the blinds or curtains and simply let the person be naked. Others get clothes that are hard for the person to remove—long dresses or robes for women, pants fixed up with suspenders at the back for men. You might find an all-in-one sweat outfit that would be hard for your aunt to take off. These are also soft and comfortable to wear. Clothing made for the disabled (the kind that is fastened at the back instead of the front) could be useful. You could probably adapt some clothes so that they have extra zippers and fastenings, some of which you could secure with a tiny padlock or pin.

If disrobing seems shocking, remember that it really is only a social embarrassment and possibly a minor legal offense. If you have visitors who might be shocked, try confining your aunt to some other room while the visitors are there. Or enlist the help of your visitors by explaining the situation to them, since they are likely to have compassion and understanding.

Violence

Q: My mother's looking after Daddy at home. He gets violent at night now and I want her to put him in the dementia unit, but she won't do it yet. Can we get the doctor to give him something to calm him down in the meantime? I'm afraid he'll hurt my mother, though he was always the sweetest, kindest man before he got Alzheimer's. What is it that makes a gentle, mellow man like my father act out so violently?

A: A lot of people, including many doctors, would say it was Alzheimer's disease, but I have to disagree.

In one sense, it is undoubtedly the fact of Alzheimer's disease that sets up the framework which contains this violence. However, it is the feelings of the person with dementia that lead to the acting out of violent episodes.

The most common feeling is fear, which comes about in reaction to something in the environment by which the person feels threatened. For example, in the care facility, such episodes most typically occur in connection with showering. This is because the resident feels extremely threatened when an invasive stranger wants to enter what was once a private situation—taking a shower—and physically carries out threatening tasks, like undressing, washing, and so on.

At home, such situations typically occur when the caregiver is trying to make the person with dementia do something that is misunderstood or, on a more global scale, when the whole atmosphere is poisoned by secrecy and lies.

I am certainly not fingerpointing or accusing when I say this, only trying to examine a complex interaction that leads to violence, so that families can unravel it. Neither am I faulting concerned family members, only highlighting the necessary skills that will make life more peaceful.

Typically the fear arises out of secrecy around Alzheimer's and mishandling of that fear. For example, when a wife sees her husband become agitated, she moves forward to soothe him. However, a man frightened enough to turn to rage needs space, not soothing. A better way to handle his anger is to stand back and let him be. Shutting men in, locking them up, or struggling hand to hand will inevitably lead to violence.

The peaceful way is to back off, to apologize for the intrusion or intervention, and to let the person come to himself again (it is most commonly men who are physically violent in cases of dementia).

Wandering

Q: *My wife slips out of the house whenever my back is turned. I can't lock her in. What can I do?*

A: Wandering is the nightmare of every caregiver and the most common problem mentioned by caregivers. That does not mean it is the most common occurrence in Alzheimer's, since by no means does everyone become a wanderer.

It is easy to see why it causes so much concern. A person who has Alzheimer's may be unable to find his or her way home and could be missing for days. Others may lack judgment about walking across highways and put themselves into grave physical danger.

The first important thing to do is to make sure that, if a person with Alzheimer's does wander away, the person carries some identifying item. You need to know when your wife leaves home, so install an alarm or bell on the door. You may add extra locks to frustrate her, but this might make her angry or upset, and there is always the chance of danger if there should be a fire and you need to exit quickly. A slip-lock placed extra high or extra low works well as a safe deterrent.

One man reports great success with painting grill-like stripes on the floor in front of the door. His wife, with the distorted perception common to Alzheimer's, refuses to step on them because she suspects that they are bars she might fall through. Another family painted a big red STOP sign on the inside of their front door and this reminded their mother not to leave the house.

The second step is to understand what is going on. It is essential for their emotional welfare that Alzheimer's patients have the freedom to move about safely. They need to get out and about for exercise and stimulation. Most people are ready for a walk when they try to leave. Take your wife for walks two or three times a day. If you can't, get someone to do so and help give your wife a sense of freedom. A high school student could do this, and your wife would have a greater sense of personal welfare if she gets some exercise and spends time outside.

All respite program and day-care centers should be able to offer safe walking for their participants, and no family should ever consider placing their family in the care of an institution that does not support safe walking for their residents.

"Safe" refers to freedom to walk within secured confines.

This chapter has covered some of the most usual problems raised by families and care staff, but people with dementia can always—and will—invent interesting new problems. Good caregivers always need to be something between a good detective and an indulgent mother when it comes to problems. Try using the three-point plan as a way of exploring those especially challenging problems.

Chapter 8

Help from
Alternative Medicine

Currently, the standard medical line on Alzheimer's seems to
be that there is nothing nonmedical people can do to help
those we care for, except to wait for a cure. This leaves most people
helpless and despairing. My experience in countrywide education
sessions is that people have been strongly discouraged from taking
matters into their own hands, even though medicine has nothing
else to offer them.

Neither have caregivers been encouraged to deal with their
own dysfunctional attitudes and to change themselves in emotional and spiritual ways that will help them cope in a better way.
It is almost disapproved of to suggest that it is time to bring
healthy caregiving into the Alzheimer's world. Well, it is time. It
is very important for all caregivers to know that we can learn better ways to cope, that we can develop and grow even with the burden of caregiving.

Alternative medicine is one avenue with much useful input
into Alzheimer's care, both in the home and in institutions. Go
ahead and investigate this area. Just remember that Hippocratic
oath we should all swear. First, do no harm. Then do some good.

Since medicine will not tell you what to look for, it is up to you
to explore for yourself. Look at possibilities in herbal medicine,
homeopathy, Chinese medicine, and dietary supplements, all of

which offer approaches to help keep people with Alzheimer's more functional within their disease.

Q: Will alternative therapies cure my mother's Alzheimer's symptoms?

A: Like medicine, alternative therapies offer no cures to Alzheimer's. What they can do is help alleviate the distress, sometimes ease the symptoms, and often improve the quality of daily life.

When seeking out alternative therapies, look for remedies that act in the following ways:
- reduce inflammation, especially in the brain
- remove toxicity from the body
- reduce stress without introducing new toxic chemicals
- improve vascular flow, especially to the brain
- improve the chemical messenger system of the brain without introducing new toxic chemicals

You must be very cautious about:
- remedies untested by time
- new fashions based on only one report (like the melatonin issue)
- medications newly approved by the Food and Drug Administration, which may prove to be inadequately tested and have toxic side effects that could be irreversible
- exploratory and experimental medications, which are even less tested and possibly more toxic; desperate families can cast caution to the wind when dealing with Alzheimer's.

Be especially cautious when dealing with approaches that are based only on statistical data that may be erroneously interpreted: for example, the claim that taking ibuprofen reduces one's chances of getting Alzheimer's. This is based on a report that concluded that people taking ibuprofen for arthritis had less incidence of Alzheimer's than the general population. Sounds good, doesn't it? However, here's something to think about: Suppose that each individual has one major stress ailment that develops with aging, so that those whose ailment is arthritis do not develop Alzheimer's.

Another claim is that taking estrogen dramatically reduces a woman's risk of developing Alzheimer's. Let's set aside the question of whether estrogen levels were ever meant to be maintained at potential child production levels for a woman's whole lifetime and what that newly introduced imbalance is likely to do to the system. Let's consider this issue: Is it estrogen itself that is important? Or is the kind of woman who is willing to take estrogen also likely to exercise, to be more involved with life, more active, more willing to learn how to deal with stress?

Q: Exactly what types of alternative medicine are helpful for someone with Alzheimer's?

A: Some of the following items can be helpful to someone you care for who has Alzheimer's or a similar dementia. *These are not prescriptions or treatments.* However, you are free to try any of them, provided that you carefully follow any indicators or limits.

If any item helps at all, do *NOT* increase dosage. More is not better. All remedies have the potential to cause harm in excess, except for homeopathy, and there is no point in increasing homeopathic intake since doing so does not increase its efficacy.

Some of these items have been endorsed by European medical experts. Others derive from other systems of medicine, such as homeopathy, herbal medicine, or Chinese medicine. Anything that I have seen mentioned as useful or significant is included; see also the list of references in the Bibliography. It is very likely that your doctor will not be familiar with these reports.

Since real knowledge is desperately lacking, please be sure to keep a journal of usage in which you faithfully record dates, dosage or amount, and any response you observe. Responses include personal opinions expressed by the person with Alzheimer's as well as whatever you notice.

Above all, be very responsible about the ways in which you use any of these items.

Herbal Medicine

Garlic

Garlic has a long history, now confirmed by modern medical research, of having an antibacterial action, as well as being a blood cleanser and a vascular stimulant. A few studies have suggested that ingestion of garlic can boost the vascular system and decrease the level of cholesterol in the body.

One of the side effects of Alzheimer's disease is decreased circulation of blood and therefore lack of oxygen to the brain. A certain amount of inflammation has also been observed in the brain tissue of people with Alzheimer's, and garlic is additionally an anti-inflammatory agent. Therefore, you might try adding garlic to the diet or using garlic pills.

Ginkgo Biloba

The Chinese have been using ginkgo and documenting its properties for at least three thousand years. Many Americans are now taking ginkgo biloba extract, but few American institutions have carried out research into its possible uses.

Hundreds of studies have been carried out in Europe by leading research institutions in France, Germany, Britain, Italy, and the Netherlands. In Germany and Italy ginkgo is licensed for the treatment of cerebral insufficiency, particularly with reference to vascular problems.

Current European research documents the wide-ranging and complex effects of ginkgo. It is considered to increase blood circulation and oxygenation of the brain, heart, eyes, ears, and limbs. Scientists relate these results to ginkgo's ability to deal with free radicals, the broken cell particles considered to be responsible for most of the effects of aging and organic degeneration.

Insufficient blood flow to the brain shows up in Alzheimer's brain scans as a major problem. Clinical experiments demonstrate that ginkgo brings about considerable improvement of blood flow in patients with cardiovascular disease. This flow goes to the healthy part of the brain but actually increases as it reaches the diseased parts of the brain. This suggests that ginkgo—like ginseng and other items from the Chinese materia medica—is an adaptogen. That is, it responds differently to the specific and varied needs of the organism.

Studies show improved memory and cognitive function in subjects taking ginkgo and good results when it is used to treat cerebral insufficiency. The symptoms of cerebral insufficiency can include inability to concentrate, memory problems, absentmindedness, confusion, lethargy, depression, anxiety, dizziness, ringing in the ears, and headaches. Ginkgo also shows good results in improvement of circulation to the legs.

A review in the prestigious British medical journal *Lancet* examined forty studies carried out with ginkgo, commending its use in the earlier stages of conditions showing cerebral insufficiency.

The Department of Geriatric Medicine, Whittington Hospital, London, confirmed cognitive improvement in their patients given ginkgo. A French study of 165 individuals showed that those most adversely affected by cerebral disorders due to aging did best on ginkgo. In three months significant improvement was noted. This would seem to indicate that ginkgo has uses in maintaining a healthy brain and body.

Perhaps ginkgo might usefully be given to people in the earlier stages of Alzheimer's. It is unknown whether it can prevent further degeneration, and it is certainly not suggested at this stage that it can cure dementia.

There are no known adverse drug reactions with ginkgo and no known side effects of ginkgo itself.

In most trials, 120–160 milligrams a day were taken, divided into three doses. There is no indication that higher amounts would serve any useful purpose.

Gotu Kola

The herb Gotu Kola originated in India but has now become part of the available Western herbal pharmacopoeia and can be found in most stores that carry herbs and natural healing nutrients.

Among its properties is its power as a vascular agent, and Christine Northrup, M.D., recommends this as part of any brain nutrition plan. For poor memory and concentration, the recommended dose is tincture taken thirty drops in water three times a day.

Ginseng

Ginseng has been used in China since at least 1000 B.C. and has become part of the standard Western herbal repertoire. It is regarded as a powerful general tonic, particularly helpful for the elderly. Research has shown that ginseng can be helpful in maintaining brain function by balancing the chemistry of the brain.

Dr. Dharma Singh Khalsa, author of *Brain Longevity*, states that Alzheimer's disease can be slowed down by the use of a number of brain nutrients, among them ginseng. His studies have revealed that Siberian ginseng seems to be the most useful for improving cognitive function and recommends 750–1,500 milligrams per day taken in capsule form. He also recommends that, instead of capsules, ginseng can be taken in the form of the patent Chinese medicine Ching Chun Bao, taking four to eight pills a day. Do not exceed doses since it can be overstimulating.

Green Tea

Green tea can be bought in all good tea stores, as well as from Japanese, Chinese, and Korean specialty stores and many health food stores. It has excellent antioxidant qualities and helps to detoxify liver and kidneys, all of which helps brain function to be improved.

Vitamins

Most dietary experts agree that elders in today's society are generally vitamin-deficient. Various studies have confirmed the seriousness of this situation, even among elders who are actually living in long-term care where one hopes that their nutritional needs are being taken care of.

Although doctors commonly say that we get all our necessary nutrition from the foods we eat and that supplements are not necessary, this has not been true since the industrialization of food production. Most people are vitamin-deficient, and this is especially serious for elders since it is directly connected with cognitive and memory problems.

Among the necessary supplements suggested by most nutrition experts for elders are the following:

Vitamin A: 25,000 units with 15 milligrams of betacarotene.

B vitamins: the four important brain nutrients are B1, B6, B12, and folic acid.

- B1 (thiamine) is vital for good brain function and daily dose should be 50–100 milligrams;
- B6 is vital for cognitive function but aging causes decline in metabolizing this vitamin, which has been shown to improve memory and circulation in a daily dose of 100mg;
- B12 helps memory, reasoning, cognitive skills, and mood control, yet it tends to be deficient in about 25 percent of elders age sixty and over, and up to 40 percent of elders over eighty. Daily dose should be 100–1,000 micrograms.
- Folic acid can enhance cerebral circulation. Low levels of folic acid seem to be related to depression and psychiatric symptoms in the elderly. One study showed that low levels of folic acid increase the likelihood of dementia by 300 percent. Daily dose should be 400 micrograms.

Vitamin C is vital for good health and especially for good brain health, yet most elders are seriously deficient in it. It is regarded as one of the most hopeful compounds for preventing Alzheimer's disease and can help even the already demented to function better and experience better general health. Take up to 3,000 milligrams a day, staggered through the day in 1,000-milligram doses.

Vitamin E is already noted for its aid in helping people resist Alzheimer's disease and even for slowing down the disease in those who already have it. Take 400 units a day, but if you are on anticoagulant drugs, check first with your doctor.

Minerals

It has been established that many people with Alzheimer's have low levels of magnesium and toxic levels of calcium in the brain. (This suggests that taking extra calcium may not be a good idea.)

Taking a supplement of 200–300 milligrams of magnesium daily helps to maintain the balance between the two. Stress of any kind depletes magnesium supplies in the system and people with Alzheimer's—who already suffer magnesium deficiency—are very stressed.

Selenium is a powerful antioxidant and an immune booster. Most elders have a deficiency of selenium and could use 50–100 micrograms daily. In the higher doses, Dr. Khalsa comments, selenium may have an anti-anxiety effect.

Zinc is considered to have an anti-aging effect, and yet, again, many people over fifty have a zinc deficiency. It helps the brain to protect itself from damage and should be taken in one 30–50 milligram dose daily.

Homeopathy

The system of homeopathic medicine was founded by the German physician Samuel Hahnemann in the 1700s. It is used all over the world today, including in the United States, where a number of M.D.s are also homeopaths.

The system is based on the idea that "like cures like." Dr. Hahnemann studied extensively and discovered that tiny amounts of certain substances—herbs, minerals, and even poisons—would stimulate the body to heal the symptoms that an overdose of the same substance would cause. Vaccines work on the same principle.

From this, he worked out a system in which a multiplicity of symptoms could be treated using the homeopathic remedies in quantities so small that some of them were virtually molecular. There are millions of users of homeopathy in the world today.

Numbers of users in the United States and all over the world are increasing.

Homeopathic remedies are available from health food stores, sometimes from pharmacies, from alternative health providers, as well as from M.D.s who prescribe homeopathically. Nearly all homeopathic remedies are available without prescription and they have no side effects.

Homeopaths acknowledge the importance of mind and body together and take into account the whole picture of symptoms, never treating only one symptom.

This holistic approach is similar to the practice of Chinese medicine, which never treats a disease but treats the whole body system as a unit. Many books can tell you much more about each system.

Q: What would be an example of homeopathic remedies for, say, my wife's memory problems?

A: Below are the homeopathic remedies that are listed in the standard homeopathic materia medica as possibilities for dealing with memory problems.

The purpose of mentioning each remedy here is to introduce you to another form of exploration, one that has been largely ignored in the United States.

You select a remedy by adding together a number of symptoms and reading a typical description of the person who has such symptoms, then finding which remedy is indicated.

Usually you will find that not all the symptoms or personal traits listed are present. This is not necessarily significant as long as the majority accurately describe the person you care for.

This description of both illness and person together indicates the body-mind-disease holistic approach of homeopathy. You are looking for a remedy for a particular person, not for an impersonal symptom.

For each remedy listed below, the first word is the name of the remedy; the number tells you what potency to use (homeopathic doses commonly come in 3X, 6X, 12X, and 30X potencies).

Those taking a homeopathic remedy should not drink coffee. Also, the medicine should not be kept near camphor or any other scented substance. When taking the tiny sugar-coated pills, do not touch the pellets with your hands. Tip them into the top of the vial and drop them under the tongue. They should not be chewed, but allowed to dissolve. No food or drink should be taken within fifteen minutes before and after the dose. Continue the medicine for one month and keep an eye on any changes.

Be aware that sometimes an intensification of symptoms is seen before improvement. This is known as the healing crisis. It is actually a good sign.

If a remedy is not useful for your family member, you will see no change for better or worse.

1. *Anacardium*, 3X every four hours for memory loss or weak memory. Indications: nervousness, irritability; low self-confidence; dyspepsia that is relieved by eating; one who walks a lot, one who is easily offended; a grumbling stomach; hemorrhoids; heart palpitations; stiff neck; skin problems; sleeplessness.

2. *Sulphur*, 6X every four hours for memory loss, especially associated with words and names. Indications: extreme forgetfulness; irritability; selfishness; depression; thinness; weakness; headaches; eye inflammations; skin problems; deafness; drinking much and eating little; frequent urination, especially at night; one who wants windows open; trembling of hands; rheumatism; one who is poor at walking; one who likes dry, warm weather.

3. *Baryta carb*, 6X every four hours for memory problems that seem like absentmindedness and inattentiveness, together with heavy, listless moods. This is a slow-acting remedy that can be repeated. Indications: hair loss; photophobia; difficulty hearing, dry mouth; catching cold easily; pain after eating, worse after consuming warm food; dry cough that worsens with change in weather; cold, clammy feet; pain in joints; twitching in sleep.

4. *Zinc*, 6X every four hours (this is homeopathic zinc, not

capsules or pills) for memory problems with a sleepy mental attitude as if thinking were hard to do. Indications: sensitivity to noise; lethargy; watering eyes; bleeding gums; heartburn from sweet food; one who is a greedy eater; involuntary urination when walking, coughing, or sneezing; small, hard, constipated stool; hoarseness; asthmatic bronchitis; one who cannot bear to be touched on the back; lameness; stepping with the entire sole of the foot on the floor; varicose veins; night sweats.

5. *Cocculus*, 3X every four hours for memory problems associated with anxiety and distraction. Indications: one who is absorbed in the imagination; sick headaches; prone to travel sickness; stomach cramps during and after meals; constant drowsiness; low fevers of nervous origin.

6. *Digitalis*, 3X every four hours for memory problems associated with finding thinking difficult to do. Indications: despondency and fearfulness; eye problems like detachment of the retina or swelling of the eyelids; discomfort after eating even a small quantity of food; enlarged, sore liver; whitish stools; deep sighing; weakness in the chest; heart palpitations caused by even the least movement; swelling of feet; fingers go to sleep.

7. *Ethusa cynapium*, 6X every four hours for memory problems associated with inability to fix one's attention. Indications: restlessness and anxiety; photophobia; a puffy face and anxious expression; milk intolerance; dry mouth; colic; undigested stools; difficulty breathing; walking or sitting with fingers and thumbs clenched.

8. *Rhododendron*, 3X every four hours for memory problems in losing a train of thought while talking. Indications: fear of thunder; hearing problems that tend to be better in the morning; toothache in damp weather; frequent breathlessness; widespread rheumatism.

You will notice that different kinds of memory problems have different homeopathic remedies indicated. People with Alzheimer's manifest various forms of memory impairment.

Homeopathy is widely used in Europe. The British royal family has a homeopathic physician in attendance. Two-thirds of all M.D.s in Germany routinely write homeopathic prescriptions. In France, doctors at the Advanced Technology Medical Center in Epinay-sur-Seine have devised a homeopathic remedy that is being widely tested on people with short-term memory problems and cognitive difficulties. Ingredients in the formula include magnesia muriatica, magnesia phosphorica, plumbum metallicum, kali phosphoricum, ambra grisea, and ginkgo biloba. Used on two groups of patients, one group of 60 and the other of 200, over 80 percent reported that they felt better or functioned better.

Unfortunately, this formula has not been put into one basic remedy by any of the homeopathic manufacturers in this country, so you would have to buy each ingredient individually and then add ginkgo, which is not a homeopathic remedy. Apart from the tediousness of having to do this, it is still workable from an exploration point of view.

Homeopathic remedies can be taken safely while any usual medications are taken for other conditions.

Aromatherapy

Q: I've heard that lavender oil seems to have a calming effect on people with Alzheimer's who get agitated. Are there other similar scents that can relieve Alzheimer symptoms?

A: Aromatherapy is yet another of those so-called New Age interests which, like Chinese medicine and homeopathy, turn out to have a long history indeed. Humankind has used oils therapeutically for about three thousand years.

It is coming back into mainstream use, for two reasons. One is that it works effectively without toxic effects, provided you follow directions and know your oils; the second is that modern medicine has begun to incorporate aromatherapy into the medical repertoire.

The interesting thing about essential oils is that their scent, although delightful, has nothing to do with their effectiveness. People with dementia usually have no sense of smell, with few exceptions. Yet they clearly respond to the therapeutic influence of oils. It is the direct response of the brain itself, not the nose, which essential oils evoke.

Different oils have different effects. Excellent books are available to help you select one for your needs. A few essential oils are especially useful in the household or institution dealing with dementia. Oils can be rubbed into the skin, sprayed in a water-oil mixture, or diffused in a room using any of several methods of diffusion.

The spray is easy and cheap, and room diffusion is the most effective. Also consider adding a few drops of oil to a hot or warm bath so it can be soaked in and breathed in. You can buy essential oils in many pharmacies, health food stores, beauty supply stores, and New Age shops.

Lavender

This is a very important resource for the home or institution dealing with dementia. It is calming and soothing without being sedating and evokes a feeling of relaxed contentment.

In a hospital in Leicester, England, a ward full of elders, many with dementia, were taken off all sleeping medications within three weeks of lavender oil being diffused throughout the night. Thereafter, lavender essential oil was all that was needed to help the elders relax, sleep well, and stay calm.

I recommended its use to a dementia unit in Newport, Oregon, near my home, and the staff reported that they noticed behavioral differences in their residents within the first two hours of using it. People were calmer, less stressed, less agitated.

It can be used day or night. If you want to keep the scent around your home, two drops of lavender oil on a kitchen cloth will clean countertops of all bacteria. A couple of drops on a fabric softener thrown in the dryer with your laundry will lightly scent all your clothes. It's great for sheets and bed linen, also to help you or the person you look after sleep better.

Orange (or lemon or lime)

Citrus oil can be used either with lavender or by itself as a mood enhancer, especially in the morning when we probably all need some extra energy.

Geranium

A light, sweet scent that helps to ease anxiety and to lift depression. It also seems to balance the hormonal system and to relieve negative moods.

If you want to use only one oil, pick lavender. You can get special diffusers for your car, for your house, and to put on a lamp.

Diet and Exercise

Q: Are there any simple things I can do that are not necessarily alternative medicine?

A: Good diet and exercise habits are universally known to promote health and well-being and to help in the prevention of disease.

Many elders suffer from malnutrition due to poor eating habits, and thus it would be wise to consider the diet of anyone suffering from Alzheimer's and to boost their system with the judicious use of vitamins.

A number of researchers suggest that general toxicity may be a big problem in the lives of people with dementia and that therefore organic foods and a balanced diet would help. Certainly, the use of caffeine and sugars probably should be limited. But since many elders are depressed, probably coffee with caffeine should be kept in the diet if the person is used to it. It has been noted to give a mood lift to the depressed.

You should avoid as much as possible:
- food additives
- food dyes
- preservatives
- foods that are almost all chemical ingredients

As one friend put it, "I don't eat anything that ends in *-ate, -ide,* or *-odium!*" Get as much natural food as possible, cut out the sodas and soft drinks and instead use water and real fruit juices.

Exercise has been proven over and over to help elders keep well if they are well, get better if they're not well, and do better even in dementia.

Walking is the easiest form of exercise, but yoga and tai chi have both been shown to help people feel better.

Chapter 9

Is Anybody Home? The Inner Journey of Alzheimer's

The caregiver's journey is one of coping and changing to meet the needs of the person with Alzheimer's, but this chapter attempts to shed some light on the inner journey of Alzheimer's.

We have often heard people with Alzheimer's described as losing their sense of self, but this does not seem to be an accurate description of what happens to most people. Very few people forget their own names, although this is not completely unheard of, and very few people lose all their memories, especially their early ones.

Q: People are so cruel about Alzheimer's. I read what they said about President Reagan. Do you think it's really true that people with this disease are empty shells?

A: Of course they aren't. This assumption gives us an excuse to avoid these people and to ignore the pain and terror around this illness. Far from being empty shells, an internal processing occurs within those affected by Alzheimer's.

There is clear evidence that most people with Alzheimer's are working through their life and memories. They are doing in Alzheimer's what most people do outside Alzheimer's. Most people, especially most older people, go through a process of reexamining their early lives and experiences—especially the issues of primal relationships and childhood experience—in order to come to some sort of resolution. Among elders, even those without specific religious affiliation, this is a spiritual process of reconciliation.

Many people in old age have reported to me that they experience memory intensification, sudden moments when total recall of an incident suddenly returns. The recall may be very vivid, including details of who was there, what they looked like, and what was said. Although this phenomenon seems to have been little reported, my experience suggests it may be widespread.

This is undoubtedly what is going on for the person with Alzheimer's, who has such an intensity of recall upon occasion—but forgets that this is only a memory and therefore enters the moment as reality. It is a flashback to a past experience, without the anchor of time orientation to remind the person this is merely memory.

Such memories are part of the process of reconciliation that goes on throughout old age up to the moment of death.

Q: My mother obviously thinks I'm her mother sometimes. She seems to want to talk about unhappy things. Is that bad for her? I don't want her getting upset.

A: By all means, encourage her to talk. This is what she needs to do. Don't worry about upsetting her. You won't. Something did upset her long ago and she needs to unload all that now so she can find peace. Be your loving self and know that you're helping her just by caring and being attentive. She'll do the rest. If she needs to cry, simply hand her tissues. Crying is good for everyone. It carries toxins out of the body and allows a person to move on emotionally instead of being stuck.

People with Alzheimer's *enter* their memory zones, rather than recall that they are memories. We could be doing a great deal more to support this process of resolution. Let us examine more fully this process, since people with Alzheimer's have for years been giving us information about it, which we have so far almost totally ignored.

There are several major themes to this process, all of which are themes that involve every human being on the great and puzzling human journey. These great human themes include: parents, childhood, belonging, home, trauma, pain, loss, meaning, dying and death, and, of course, the greatest of all human themes—the search for love. These are exactly the themes that are constantly being explored by people with Alzheimer's. In fact, having Alzheimer's disease in no way interferes with the process of exploring these great life themes, although it may lead to them being worked on at a more intuitive rather than rational level.

People with Alzheimer's are constantly working on these themes, are always talking about them to anyone who will listen or talking to themselves in the absence of anyone else to interact with. They urgently need our support to continue and validate the process so as to reach personal peace. Once we understand that this profound process is going on, even within an impaired person, we can see our own task of caring for people with Alzheimer's as a very different one. Not only does it give them the respect from us that they deserve, but it helps us as their care-givers.

This process changes our role from the custodial one, which is wearing us all down and destroying people with Alzheimer's with the sterility we inflict on them, to the much more honorable role of assisting the person to make peace on a very deep level.

Q: I work in a special care unit as an aide. I have ten people to look after, and I often get the feeling they need more from me than I'm giving. Do you have any ideas what they need?

A: I certainly do, but I don't know if you'll be allowed to meet their needs in the traditional medical model of care. However, I do want to thank you for caring, since I know your residents will sense your concern.

To reassess the way in which we work with people with Alzheimer's will require a major series of attitude changes among those who currently control how such work is done. It is not un-common to find that many of those working with people with de-mentia are task-oriented, rather than person-oriented.

This means they may regard a successful day as one in which everyone was washed, put on clean clothes, and got fed—some-thing we might classify as the "pet rabbit" syndrome. "Pet rabbit" care tends to typify much of what we are currently doing for people with dementia. It offers the necessary basic physical care but neglects the nurturing of the spirit and support of the person that individuals really need. We undoubtedly underestimate those with dementia.

This probably has everything to do with the withdrawal, loss of personhood, and decline that we currently think of as the disease process. It might be truer to classify these losses as "care dam-age"—an adult version of the failure to thrive that has been found among infants in institutional care where the need for con-tact, love, and personal interaction has been neglected.

Q: You talk about the journey people are on, but what is that journey? How do we know what that process is?

A: How do people with Alzheimer's present the classical themes of their inner processes? Obviously, they do it somewhat differently from people who do not have dementia. For one thing, they are much more caught up in the dynamic of the process, since they are not distanced by intellectual information about time zones, calendar limitations, and a continuing division between past and present. They are often caught up in the exis-tential continuous present, where Mother is coming home and Father has gone to work.

These intellectual shortfalls in no way invalidate the worth or achievement of their psychological processing, however. Neither do they make any statements about the validity of what those with Alzheimer's undergo.

Q: My mother thinks her daddy is coming to get her. The doctor says she's hallucinating. Does this means she's crazy?

A: No, I don't believe that applying the word *hallucination* to her emotional experiences is useful or even accurate. We have been slow to apply the word *flashback* to such experiences.

Using jargon from the psychiatric world—*hallucination* or *delusion*, for example—implies a pathological symptom rather than a meaningful process. Given that much of Alzheimer's disease is undoubtedly severely stressful—and that this disease often seems to come into a life already extremely stressed—perhaps we should be looking toward the vocabulary of stress-related processes.

Flashbacks, posttraumatic stress syndrome, and so on are more appropriate terms rather than psychiatric labels from the world of mental illness. We might even usefully employ the term *extreme state* for Alzheimer's disease to remind ourselves that it is not a mental illness, but rather a process or set of processes reflecting lifetime issues, even if contained within the framework of dementia. The classic themes of the Alzheimer's journey are as follows.

Parents

The theme of primary relationships exists whether or not the person actually knew his or her parents, just as it does for all of us. It has a denotative meaning through the early events of our lives and parental experiences, but it also has a symbolic and emotional meaning related to our inner feelings at any given time.

"Sometimes I feel like a motherless child," goes the great Negro spiritual, and it is a feeling that has undoubtedly swept over most human beings at one time or another when they feel particularly lost, unnurtured, and unhappy. That yearning to feel like a mothered child is a human archetype.

If, for whatever reason, we are insufficiently parented and nurtured, then we deal with the theme of orphanhood. Orphanhood is also a parent theme, as are abandonment, abuse, and loss of parenting. It might be more accurate to call this issue "mothering" rather than parenting.

To know where a person with Alzheimer's is in dealing with this theme, we need only listen to what is said.

"When are my mother and father coming home to dinner?" asks the eighty-seven-year-old woman, in her own home, who had lived with her parents until their deaths at advanced ages.

"Where is my mother? I haven't seen her for so long, I just can't stand it," says a ninety-year-old woman, recently moved into a care center, who then collapses into a torrent of weeping.

"My daddy hurt my mom and he's trying to hurt me," says a frightened little woman of seventy-nine years, also in a care facility.

In part, it would be correct to regard these remarks as echoes from former life habits, but there is more going on in the person than that. Each of the statements tell us that these women are involved with the need, the yearning—and, in the third case, the fear—still working in their lives around parental issues.

We need to respect this process, because we all do it. We all have parents living forever inside our hearts and minds, long after they are dead. We often live lives that echo the roles our parents played in our own being in the world. The only difference is that people with Alzheimer's reveal themselves more nakedly.

This is why we have been so wrong to regard Alzheimer's as a disease that strips away personhood. It strips the person of concealment, often revealing a hitherto unknown human being to family members and spouses. What then should our responses be to statements and questions regarding parents?

The answer requires a sensitive reading of the situation. The response called for is seldom a rational one. We need to sensitize everyone who works with people with Alzheimer's not to torment them with rational replies that do not meet their needs.

"Where is my mother?" does not call for the rational response, "She's dead."

After all, when a wounded soldier cries out for his mother, we do not insist on orienting him to the fact that his mother is actually six thousand miles away. We recognize the emotional need in his question. We should not be so reluctant to recognize the emotional needs of those wounded first by Alzheimer's and then by the failures of our care institutions.

Clearly, the person asking for a parent is at that moment *feeling* motherless, and this is a message that some nurturing action would be appropriate—a hug, a cup of coffee, a walk.

To the staff member who says there is no time for all this, the answer is that families are paying for appropriate care and this *is* appropriate Alzheimer's care. "Pet rabbit" care is not appropriate, and the time is not far off when families are going to start demanding some changes in standards of the expensive care they are paying for.

Childhood

Q: *My pop keeps telling us about his brother, who drowned in front of his eyes when he was ten. Then he'll cry and we feel awful too. Is there some way to deal with this that will stop him dwelling on bad stuff?*

A: Your father is already dealing with it and all he really needs is your ears.

Childhood is the most powerfully affecting time of our lives, the one that all of us have to work and rework until everything is resolved. Often people repeat a traumatic event over and over, and all that is needed from us is a sympathetic response: "That's terrible." "That must have been awful!" "I'm really sorry that it happened," and so on.

The person will continue to repeat this trauma until it is no longer an issue—which may be never. Those who work with people with Alzheimer's should not feel they have failed when these stories continue to be repeated. Neither should they assume the stories are repeated because of memory problems. They are repeated because the trauma is still echoing within. The kindest thing we can do is to listen as if it were the first time.

Home and Sense of Belonging

Q: My husband wants me to take him home but we are home, so I don't know how to help him.

A: Often intertwined with the issues of childhood is the companion issue of home. For all human beings, home is more than a place. It is an archetype containing multiple ideas: a sense of belonging, a sense of safety, a sense of being loved and cared for, and a sense of the known and the familiar. Even if an individual did not experience these actual events at home, or never had a home, a longing for home still exists within the human psyche.

This is especially true in those with Alzheimer's disease who are constantly being challenged on the issues of belonging and safety. Often they have actually been displaced from their familiar home; even if they have not, the disease itself tends to displace them by making the familiar unfamiliar. In fact, it might be correct to say that having Alzheimer's disease means never being at home anymore. So, at the point at which the person is sorting through this great issue, actual home is being lost.

Often, if those with Alzheimer's are in care facilities, the staff tend to assume that the home to which they refer is the one they have previously lived in, but this is no more likely to be true than if they were living at home. People still in their homes will ask to go home, just like your husband. Obviously, this refers to some other place than the one they are in. By paying attention, we can begin to comprehend what "home" is in the Alzheimer's theme.

It is time-place-person, a complexity of elements that we might best describe as "homeness." It usually refers to the past and most often to childhood, though not necessarily. It is a nostalgia that cannot be re-created, no matter how families try.

One kind but misguided family in California took their father back to San Antonio because he kept telling them he wanted to go home. When they got there, however, they found he wanted San Antonio in 1926—he was horrified by the San Antonio of the 1990s.

Knowing that this is a profound issue for those with dementia, we should be addressing the question of how we propose to create a sense of homeness for those we care for.

Trauma

Q. We never knew all the family secrets until Mom got sick. Then it all came tumbling out of her. Is this because of her dementia?

A: Past trauma is often a theme of people with dementia, frequently in the form of repetitive story, and our task is simply to listen and respond appropriately each time we hear it.

Sometimes caregivers ask how often they have to listen. The answer is: until the person has told the story enough—which may be a finite time or may continue until death. The person with dementia repeats stories, not because of dementia, but because of the power of the story that demands it be told.

One of the growth opportunities afforded by Alzheimer's is the removal of the suppression mechanism. This can allow formerly unspeakable things to be said. Often, however, this opening of previously unspoken material can come about only in a supportive setting. It does not happen merely because a person has dementia and does not remember to conceal secrets. An atmosphere of safety is also necessary for the process to occur.

For example, one woman in a day respite program had the following episode of unfoldment. For six weeks she had been attending the psychosocial program, in which bonding, safety, and affection were more important than the nature of the activities. All those who attended regularly gathered around a table, and interaction was facilitated tactfully by staff.

The woman, whose home situation was quite abusive, had become closely bonded with another participant and clearly felt safe with the others. On this particular day she seemed distracted and nervous, picking at a toilet paper roll on the table. She examined the toilet roll closely, turning it round and round in her hand, picking at the paper. She made several attempts to say something, broke off each time, then began again.

By this time, everyone around the table was aware that something was going on and they were watching her. She took up the toilet roll again and stared at it closely while she made another attempt to speak. This time, she was able to tell her story.

When she was about eleven years old, she had begun attending a Baptist church Sunday school. One day the pastor decided to hold a picnic for the Sunday school children. She attended the picnic. After all the children had lunch, she needed to go to the toilet and the pastor had volunteered to take her. He led the little girl by the hand to the bathroom and, once she was inside, he had sexually assaulted her. Then, in the usual modus operandi of child molesters, the pastor had warned her that she would go to hell if she ever said anything about it, because she was a bad little girl.

The woman wept painfully as she gasped out this story, and the whole group gave her strong and loving emotional support.

No one could possibly have guessed that the presence of a toilet paper roll could have triggered such a story. It serves to remind us that, indeed, we can never know what power ordinary objects carry for people. Without a setting of sufficient respect, affection, and safety, the lost stories within, the tales of old wounds, do not and cannot emerge. In a setting where such an individual would have become lost in a crowd of needy old people getting only maintenance care from overwhelmed workers, such a story would never have emerged.

Q: My mother tells about finding a severed head rolling in the waves off the coast of Hawaii during the war. Do you think this is true?

A: Of course we can't know, but studies of people with Alzheimer's have indicated they are as accurate as people without dementia when it comes to recounting tales of the past.

This means they are as accurate and as inaccurate. So, whether your mother is inventing or retelling does not matter at this point. All she needs is your listening ear and an appropriate response gauged to her emotional state when she recounts this story.

There is some purpose to the telling of the story, whatever its truth, and listening meets her need. Emotional pain seems to need a witness for the final healing to take place—a validation that helps the person leave the pain behind.

Often elders have stifled their emotional pains. Often they had no support during their hard passages in life, or they felt that they "had to be strong," or "men don't cry," which was interpreted as meaning "show no emotion." Otherwise, they were culturally unsupported in having normal human feelings.

One family reports, "Our youngest brother died at seventeen years old and no one in the family ever mentioned his name again. We two sisters were three and four years older than him and we only put a headstone on his grave when we were thirty-five and thirty-six. Our mother died without ever saying his name again, and our father spent the last week of his life deliriously calling out, 'Barry! Barry!' That was our brother's name."

This man had to wait until his deathbed before he could openly mourn his beloved son's death. Some version of this story is not at all uncommon among this generation of elders.

Sometimes the feelings at the time were so overwhelming that the person felt unable to admit them in case the pain made it impossible for life to go on. Often, however, the time never did come when the feelings could be dealt with. Once the emergency was over, the matter was pushed aside.

Often, the bereaved or hurting person will still say, "But I don't want to think about it. It's too painful." This indicates that the original pain was never dealt with.

When a society loses the rituals of death and mourning, it strands itself in a swamp of undealt-with feelings. This is what we often find in our elders. They have become stranded and it is up to those who look after them not to continue the process of being stuck.

Issues of loss often surface when people become absorbed by Alzheimer's disease, for two reasons. One is that the suppression mechanisms—which are tricks of mind, not of heart—are gradually lost; the other is that having Alzheimer's disease is such a process of loss in itself that it triggers all other previously experienced loss processes. Therefore, we can reasonably expect to see major loss issues emerge in people with dementia, and we need to recognize this as a potential source of healing, not as a negative event.

When people share this pain with us, they do not need cheering up. This does not need saying in a therapeutic setting, but in care settings it needs saying often. Care staff often have difficulty accepting that living in care is a profound loss.

The most common response is to label sorrow as depression—thus depersonalizing it by assuming it is a pathology—and to drug people, instead of accepting the grief process and facilitating its resolution.

People with dementia need to have their honest feelings—of grief, rage, and loss—without the threat of their emotions being medicated out of them. It is appropriate to mourn the loss of normal life. Those who are allowed to mourn as they need to can come to a deeper, richer sense of life or at least to acceptance.

After all, those we care for have a whole lifetime of grief, joy, pain, and pleasure to look back on, which helps them to make necessary if unwanted adjustments. They are not children. They have had experienced lives, and we can trust them to make the necessary adjustments with our respectful input wherever it might help.

Dying

Q: Lately, my father keeps saying things like, "I wish I could just go home," and he lives at home. Why does he keep repeating this?

A: Most people are afraid of dying and of death. Some are afraid of the process of dying, but not of death itself.

We can assume that the same fear is present in people with Alzheimer's disease, especially since fear is a major part of the disease process. We need to be especially alert for any references that might be overt or covert allusions to dying and to death, in order that we can respond supportively.

Often people's references to home at some point become references to death, especially in the weary soul whose day-to-day life is deeply unrewarding.

"I wish I could just go home."

"I'm ready."

"I want to be with my parents again."

All of these may be references to death; often the caregiver who knows this person best will have a sense of whether that is true. It is useful and supportive for the caregiver to respond in equally obscure yet kindly terms:

"You'll be able to go when you're ready."

"It won't be hard, you'll see."

"It's natural to be scared, but it'll be okay. Everyone does it. You'll know how, when the time comes."

Fear

Q: Is it true my husband will get angry now that he has Alzheimer's? And what about depression? I hear a lot of people get depressed and have to take pills. Is that right?

A: There is a lot to be said about the emotional journey of Alzheimer's, much of which has been ignored by those who should have been helping families understand the process.

Our ignoring, misinterpreting, and mislabeling these issues has often led to poor care, both at home by well-meaning family members and even more so in care institutions.

Partly this has come about because we have tended to exclude people with dementia from input into their own care, as if having dementia meant never knowing your own mind about anything.

It may not be entirely untrue that people have trouble knowing their own minds during this passage. However, they clearly do know their own feelings—or perhaps more accurately stated, they *experience* their own feelings. We have done little to try to understand what it is they are experiencing, although they have been demonstrating their feelings to us for years in actions and behaviors.

We should never forget that the dominant emotion in Alzheimer's disease is fear: continual, unrelenting, day-after-day terror. If anyone should doubt that, consider how terrified we as

167

a society are of this disease. Alzheimer's has virtually been demonized by society as the one most-dreaded disease, the one people most fear to have. Why should a person who actually has the disease have any less fear?

In fact, the fear is greater because the person is undergoing unimaginable losses. Everything that makes life safe, reliable, and fun is going. The sense of inner structure is going. Even the ability to have a life is going. And the ordeal starts anew each day. There is no relief. Often, even at home, this person does not get the necessary help and support.

In an institution, where all kinds of random and explicable people, events, and structures appear and disappear, that fear becomes even more intense.

It is useful for us to remember that typically, though not inevitably, men cover such fear with anger, while women cover it with anxiety or tears. Therefore, when we hear that a man is acting out his anger, we need to ask, "What scared him?" rather than labeling him "combative." When a woman cries a lot, we need to find ways to explore fear with her rather than drugging her into a sort of compliantly quiet depression.

Whatever feelings your husband has will be in response to his inner and outer world. And, no, it is not necessarily true that he must be angry or depressed.

Terminal Illness, the Kübler-Ross Way

Q: Do you think people with Alzheimer's know they have Alzheimer's, and, if they do, what does this mean for them?

A: I am entirely sure that they know, and that they continue to know it even into the deepest parts of their illness process.

In Dr. Elisabeth Kübler-Ross's groundbreaking work on death and dying, we have an excellent framework for understanding their emotional process in this terminal illness. Most professionals and many families are familiar with Kübler-Ross's unfolding of the experiences commonly undergone by the person who is suffering a terminal illness.

Through years of working in hospitals with the dying, she explored how the dying can be helped with their processes by our understanding and acceptance. She dismantled the former practice of virtually ignoring the dying and maintaining secrecy about death. She introduced instead a compassionate and insightful structure of psychological support. Unfortunately, we have not included this kind of progress in most of our attitudes toward those with Alzheimer's.

Again, it is as if we have concluded that people with dementia do not have feelings about their illness, do not notice they are ill, and anyway are not undergoing any such process.

My ten years of working with people with dementia, including those who were dying, suggests to me that the very opposite is true: those who are terminally ill with Alzheimer's go through the same processes that Kübler-Ross identified.

The stages she identified were denial, grief, anger, and, ultimately, acceptance and reconciliation with the truth of dying. Not all people go through all stages, neither do they experience them in order, nor do they necessarily go through each one only once. There may be a considerable recycling of various stages until everything has been worked through.

We have acknowledged that people with dementia get angry, feel sad, and go through denial of their illness, but we have apparently assumed that they do this meaninglessly and with no connection with real process. We seem to have made this error because of a mistaken assumption that somehow the stages identified by Kübler-Ross are rational processes made by choice. Therefore, we seem to have assumed that people with dementia could not be going through them, because their rational process and memory reliability are fracturing.

However, what Kübler-Ross identified were *emotional* processes coming from the deepest being of a person stricken with terminal illness, an organic reaction to being besieged by sickness. There is no reason to assume that people with dementia are excluded from these processes. In fact, long-term observation and interaction with them will serve to confirm they do indeed undergo these passages. We simply have not put the evidence together in a rational way, mainly because we mistakenly assume that feelings are mind-produced, whereas they are experience-produced.

A generalized prejudice exists against admitting that anything meaningful is going on within people with dementia. This seems to be no different from the generalized prejudice of thirty years ago that said that children with cerebral palsy were empty of consciousness, intelligence, and human response.

Part of such judgments comes from simply not paying enough attention to the people in our care; possibly the other part comes from our own fear of their condition. We prefer to assume they are unaware and unfeeling, rather than admit they are just like us, but struggling with a profoundly difficult journey of dysfunction.

Once we acknowledge that there are recognizable emotional processes going on within people with dementia, we can begin to help them with the appropriate support and validation.

Spiritual Issues

Q: I'm a pastor at a hospital with a special Alzheimer's wing and I would like to do more to help its residents. Some are very impaired indeed and I'm wondering how to help them.

A: Everyone has a spiritual aspect to their life whether or not he or she realizes it. It is often those without such awareness who are most prone to hopelessness and despair. This leaves us with the task of considering how we may nurture that spiritual side of their being even though they themselves do not.

Whatever else Alzheimer's may be, it is certainly a psychospiritual crisis, a state in which the individual is overwhelmed by what is happening. And the most pressing aspect of this whole crisis is the crisis of love. If there is one great issue for the individual with Alzheimer's, it is the question of love: the quest to receive unconditional love before dying, through dying, and into the process of death.

Most residents in any kind of institutional care are living in a desperate crisis of love, both conditional and unconditional. Those who care for them need to give attention to how they can create an atmosphere of unconditional love.

The central spiritual offering needed in dementia care is *relationship*. To create such a relationship, you need to give enough time for a sense of contact to be felt. Sit a while, reach out to the person, perhaps with physical touch—simply *be with* the person.

Loneliness is the greatest source of pain for residents in long-term care. So sit, talk, and make eye and heart contact, without hurried or sudden movements. Try to represent not God the Father, but the emotional and spiritual essence of God the Mother.

Q: My aunt has Alzheimer's, lives in a care home, and is mainly bedridden now. I visit as often as I can and recently she told me her father had been coming to see her at night. The woman who runs the home said my aunt has also reported visits from her brothers and sisters. All these people are dead. What is making her have these hallucinations?

A: My guess is that your aunt may be preparing for her own death. I don't find it useful to apply psychiatric jargon to these experiences, since that dismisses them as irrelevant and pathological. Many of us who work with elders know that once the dead relatives start visiting death soon follows. It is a common phenomenon among elders who are approaching death.

While we might argue about their origin—psychiatric, spiritual, brain chemistry, near death experiences—obviously we can't classify them other than in our own opinions. Therefore, I prefer to acknowledge them as a signal of imminent change.

Instead of worrying about them, become an interested party. "Oh really? What did your grandfather look like? Did he say anything?"

That approach encourages your aunt to talk about anything that might be on her mind right now.

Chapter 10

Unconditional Love

The secret to good Alzheimer's care is love. Love is the greatest resource in living with Alzheimer's disease. Apart from all its other difficulties, Alzheimer's involves a crisis of love, both on the part of the person who has the disease and on the part of all those who live with or are involved with it. The person who has Alzheimer's disease has an undisguised yearning for love and is often as open as a child to the longings of the heart. In this sense, we could say that Alzheimer's disease turns into a journey from the mind to the heart.

Q: My wife is really ill with Alzheimer's disease. She's in care now and when I go to see her, she calls me Daddy. Should I tell her I'm not her father?

A: She's naming your emotional role for her now. This is not an identification problem, though it may sound as if it is.

Typically, people with Alzheimer's express their longings for deep emotional security and unconditional love. Often, we do not choose to hear what they say. We may feel it is too painful to deal with the issues of their deep needs and human longings.

Either at home or in care situations, it is typical for these words to be dismissed as the babbling of dementia, but if we stop and listen, we can plainly hear the longings clearly expressed:

"I want to go home."

"I want to see my mother."

"I'm lonely."

"No one ever comes to see me."

These are not just nonsense or meaninglessly repeated complaints. They are the deepest longings of human beings: to be cared for and accepted, to be cherished and protected, to be loved. We are face to face with the profound human hunger for unconditional love. That can make many of us feel uncomfortable or inadequate, especially if we face at the same time our inability to really give such love.

Q: I'm worried that my stepfather is abusing my mother, who has Alzheimer's. He's very angry at her all the time and says he wants to get rid of her. They were happy for over thirty years. What's going on?

A: Many relationships are based on conditional love. In fact, they are much more common than those based on unconditional love. For example, married love may well depend on decades-long exchanges between husband and wife. These exchanges are often connected with accepting roles, carrying through perceived duties, and finding a basis for gratifications.

When one partner can no longer carry through these arrangements, a crisis of love arises. The unimpaired partner becomes impatient, angry, feels trapped because a certain sense of orderliness has been disrupted and a lifestyle thrown into chaos. This is obviously your parents' situation, whatever the reasons that might underlie it. Probably you already suspect the real reasons for their anger with each other.

You may need to step in to protect her. If she is unsafe, she needs to be moved to a safe environment, whether that is your house or a care home of some kind. Perhaps your stepfather needs more help and more support himself. I wonder if you have sat down to talk with him. He might manage better if he had time off while your mother went to a day respite program, or if he had help in the house.

Since you fear for her safety, intervene soon rather than stand by. Abuse of elders is not uncommon in this country, so you are right to want to do something. If you can't intervene directly, then notify the senior services agency or call your local elder abuse hotline.

Q: I find it really hard to have to help my own mother take showers and remind her to do things. I used to look up to her, now I just want to run away from her. Am I a monster?

A: No, you're an overworked, emotionally overburdened human being who's finding the changes in your mother hard to deal with. That's understandable. You're dealing with Alzheimer's, which is demanding enough. But you're also dealing with a major loss and change of relationship. The perceived task of a parent is to nurture, to be protective and concerned, to give unconditional love to the child, to be unchanging and faithful in the parental role. If that parent should begin instead to ask for nurturing, for protection, for a parental type of love from the child, a crisis of love arises.

It asks a great deal of you to be accepting of your change in roles. You are in the middle of this crisis of love, and you need help, time off, and perhaps some counseling to get you through it.

Don't get too caught up in the details of your mother's illness, but don't displace the issue either. The more you understand about her illness, the less you will blame her for her symptoms. Often, what family members do instead is to search for care to be given. Either the family member becomes totally involved in care on a one-on-one basis, or becomes caught up in trying to obtain that level of care in other ways: finding the right nursing home, hiring the perfect caregiver, even moving to another part of the country because the right kind of care might exist there.

Much of this desperate searching is connected with the fact that a crisis of love has arisen (or has finally been revealed), a crisis that is not being dealt with.

The person with Alzheimer's disease gives us perfect opportunities to practice unconditional love and compassion. It doesn't matter that we never asked to practice it. It doesn't matter that we never wanted to become a caregiver or that we do so reluctantly. We can still become good caregivers, making a spiritual pathway of the task and letting it be an opportunity for growth.

If we can really understand the childlike terrors that awaken an old woman in the night, instead of being impatient with being awakened ourselves, we feel compassion.

If we really comprehend the confusion of not knowing what day it is, not recognizing anyone we love, we feel tenderness and protectiveness. When this other human being appears to us unprotected and vulnerable, plainly needing our help, we are touched by that need.

Or so we might hope.

The reason we so often fail as caregivers to have this understanding and to feel this compassion is certainly not that we are bad people—far from it. If we are trying to be caregivers, we do so out of our innate goodness. We fail most often because we do not allow the time that love needs. We fill up our day with a thousand caregiving duties and demands. Many of these are really unimportant, because often we are avoiding our own inner feelings or pain. We have no sense of proportion about what matters because we forget the importance of love.

If the person you care for died tonight, would you rather say, "Well, at least his clothes got washed so I can bury him in clean ones," or, "Thank goodness we sat and held hands together while the sun went down"? The answer probably looks obvious on paper, but we often tend to forget it during the day, especially when we feel overwhelmed by demands and the tasks that need to be done.

Alzheimer's gives us unique opportunities to deal with the issues of love—unconditional, compassionate love, unattached to any expectations, any duties, any rewards other than the bliss of being in that wonderful flow for a while. None of the conditional-love pictures fit.

The person with Alzheimer's cannot be your mother if she is living in the memory of being sixteen and thinks you are her brother. The woman who is your wife cannot do the washing, cleaning, cooking, or shopping duties with any accuracy. How then will you find it in yourself to love this person?

One way is to let go of your expectation of the roles that this person used to fill and simply accept the present moment. This is very hard for most of us to do. Without even thinking about it, we are totally attached to people's usual roles.

We find it very hard to let go of our expectations. Much of our love for any particular person is attached specifically to that person's role in our life. In Alzheimer's, people forget their roles and those around them find it hard to forgive or accept. Instead, they stay attached to some other time, some other situation, never living in the now.

Yet there is no other reliable moment in Alzheimer's. The past may be forgotten, the future has no reality, but there is here and now. Being lovingly with someone in the here and now, with no past or future pictures, no conditional behavior expectations, is both very hard and extremely easy.

It is hard because we seldom give up our mental pictures of what we want from a person or what we expect or how we judge. It is hard because our minds are usually running here and there, anywhere but now. It is easy because we only have to sit there and hold hands lovingly and think and be love. It takes so little to give, but doing it is like reaching across an ocean.

A family member may be loving and accepting with a child and yet be unable to accept the same behavior in an adult. "I can accept this in my four-year-old, but not in my father-in-law," says Maureen. Yet there is no difference between the two in their need for love. The difference is in Maureen.

Q: They talk about a "cancer personality." Is there an Alzheimer's personality, someone especially likely to get Alzheimer's?

A: I believe there is. Whenever I describe this to families, they often identify their sick family member as conforming to it in significant ways.

Based on my observations of people with Alzheimer's, I would draw the following picture of the "Alzheimer's personality": someone with severe early childhood difficulties, possibly born into abusive or unnurturing family situations or into a totally dysfunctional world such as that of a concentration camp. This person lacked nurturing, was orphaned or abandoned, or had one parent absent in some way and the other unable to nurture.

Life for this person continued to be demanding, to impose a great deal of unusual stress or trauma. The person often entered into a marriage that did not meet his or her emotional needs.

Often, the person who later develops Alzheimer's has worked in a profession or job weighted with the care of other people in some way—social workers, teachers, and nurses seem to predominate. So the early lack of nurturing continues throughout life. Emotional pain and stress are never dealt with and accumulate within.

This seems particularly fitting because Alzheimer's disease involves a sense of *psychospiritual crisis*. If the crisis did not exist before—and almost invariably it did—it certainly comes about within the illness.

What is meant by the phrase *psychospiritual crisis*? It means that a person is living without inner resources, without a real inward sense of being whole, often exhausted by a lifetime in which few needs have been met. Often the crisis involves early deprivation and loss never resolved.

Psychospiritual crisis often comes about in a person who has never had the chance to become himself or herself, who has been buried in roles and the expectations of others. In a person whose system is already being overwhelmed—as in Alzheimer's disease—a complete dissolution comes about.

A survey of an Alzheimer care unit in the San Francisco Bay Area revealed that of the fifty-four people in the unit, a startlingly high number had been teachers, nurses, social workers, and caregivers. All their lives, many of the residents had given over their time to the nurturing of others. Moreover, a significant number had undergone lives of considerable crisis and deprivation, especially when they were children. Some were starved and beaten as children, raped, molested, put in concentration camps, orphaned, abandoned. Others had been abused continually as adults, had undergone treatment with psychiatric medications, had been victims of crimes of violence. The degree of drama in these lives had been markedly high.

So, aside from all the genetic and environmental factors that may be involved in this disease, it looks as if there is an inner crisis of another kind at work. We know stress underlies many conditions, why not this one?

Q: My husband is so clinging and helpless since the doctors diagnosed him with Alzheimer's. I find it hard to put up with this. Do you have any suggestions to improve our relationship, from my point of view?

A: The Chinese say wisely, "When you cannot change a situation, you have to change your mind." Since you can't change your husband or his disease, you have to change yourself so that this does not become a crisis of love for you.

Many of us love on a fairly small-scale way; that is to say, we give love for exchange, for control, for gratification, for duty, and for some inner emptiness that we seek to have filled. Unconditionally loving someone with Alzheimer's can introduce us to a much larger way of loving and can put us in touch with an entirely different set of values.

We cannot experience that as long as we are too frightened to really look at this illness. We cannot do it while we are too angry to be able to sit down and really be with the person. We cannot do it when we are so consumed by what lies within us that we cannot sit still.

If we can practice letting go, being here in the present moment, reaching out with compassion and just letting flow happen, everything gets easier.

This kind of loving is not sentimental, airy-fairy, pie-in-the-heavenly-sky stuff. It is the most practical and rewarding way to get through an Alzheimer day. Real unconditional love works. It works better than drugs or than shouting at someone or scolding, and it is an effective way of managing difficult behaviors.

Your doctor might not think of telling you to try unconditional love as a way of dealing with Alzheimer's, but as a caregiver, you will find it works. Instead of fighting to control the person, you let go and—surprise—the battle is over.

You can get someone with Alzheimer's to do what you want as soon as you stop wanting it. It is the tension of the two of you wanting that keeps the resistance up and, for example, stops your husband from being able to get his sweater on properly. Your emotional tension causes confusion and dysfunction in your husband. So, when you let go of your tension about his neediness and fear, you may find he seems less needy and fearful. Whatever you are hiding inside you will be reflected back by your husband. That is what makes Alzheimer's so uncomfortable for others to deal with. Women who were always meek and obedient to their husbands show their anger. Men who were strong, silent, take-charge types weep. Those with Alzheimer's often show us part of ourselves we do not like to deal with.

If you and your spouse are unhappy, your children will manifest unhappiness too, no matter how careful you are to be kind to them. Likewise, the person with Alzheimer's is not protected by the barriers that most of us erect against the things we do not wish to know or see. The person with Alzheimer's is very sensitive to the feelings of others.

If you can relax and lovingly be with your husband in the here and now, you will be fed by an expansion, a warmth, an exchange of deep love. You will be filled because unconditional love is not a measure, it is a flow.

Q: How do you give unconditional love when you feel angry or depressed or just plain fed-up?

A: First, unconditional love doesn't mean behaving like a perfect human being, although it might be nice to be able to be one. However, no one is perfect. Unconditional love means not losing touch with the fact that you and this person are in the same flow of eternal unchanging love, even when you feel angry.

Ready to try unconditional love?

- Sit still and do nothing. Just be.
- Take several deep breaths and resolve to set everything else aside for the moment, all the problems, resentments, uncomfortable feelings.
- Look for the yearning for love however it is expressed by that person you know so well. Does the stubborn set of the shoulders tell you this person is frightened to let his need show? Are the eyes questioning and fearful? Is the body rigidly fixed into no-one-can-ever-hurt-me toughness? Is the face an iron mask that hides all feelings? If so, what is the deepest feeling you imagine hiding behind the mask?
- Where is the child inside who never had enough love, enough care, perhaps even enough food or safety? Can you see that child at all? Can you feel compassion for that child? Did this person ever tell you about early life and its hardships?
- Can you now forgive everything you never had from this person? If you can, that will heal your own hurts because it allows you to experience unconditional love. Any time you do, it flows back in time to all your wounds and heals them.

It is appropriate to feel sad as you undergo this process of compassion. People suffer greatly in this world, and our compassion makes us feel sad for them. As we feel sad for them, we inevitably reflect back on any sadness we feel for our own suffering in this life. Most of the suffering you read and hear about in connection with Alzheimer's is not the suffering from the disease itself. It is the suffering of the family.

Q: My father was once a professor of physics at an Ivy League university, and now he's totally disabled by Alzheimer's. That magnificent mind has gone and in its place is a man who likes to play with toys and pet animals. This is driving me crazy. Is there any way to make this bearable?

A: While I'm not suggesting you forget the man your father was, it would be less painful if you could move forward into his present, where he may actually be experiencing happiness. Much family suffering circles around unwillingness to let go of the past and move into the present.

It's true that having Alzheimer's is a horrifying thing to those who don't have it—but then, being old is horrifying to the young. Being disabled is horrifying to those who are able-bodied. Many of the things we imagine would make life unbearable become things we deal with when they actually happen.

Human beings are much more resilient than we sometimes think and more attached to life than we acknowledge. We do a lot of projection on Alzheimer's, since it contains all we fear most. It would be more useful to face our own inner fears than to project them on the person with Alzheimer's.

In your case, if you imagine your father is inwardly saying, "How terrible that I've lost my magnificent mind!" you would be mistaken most of the time. He may be thinking, "These [toy] cars are neat!" You may think that's a tragedy, but that's just life for him.

Families do this often, understandably, but it creates huge gaps of connection that fill with loneliness. The way to close the gap is not to hang on to the past but simply to come forward. After all, you can still love your father and he can still feel loved. That isn't a sentimental thought; it is the only reality.

I saw this dilemma lived out often when I was a medical social worker in an Alzheimer's care unit in the San Francisco area.

"Bill would have hated to be somewhere like this," said his wife, standing in the special care unit where Bill had been placed. "His sister had Alzheimer's and he always said he'd hate to end up like her."

Actually, at that very moment, Bill was happily walking around trying to organize a group to take part in a musical activity. He was cheerful and upbeat, as he was every day without fail. The Bill who hated the idea of Alzheimer's had been forgotten and this Bill was content and busy with all kinds of self-appointed activities.

His wife, however, suffered every time she came to see him because she was still relating to that gone-away Bill. For her, he was endlessly suffering even though in his new reality he was demonstrably happy. Bill's wife was trapped in the past. In that, she was typical of many Alzheimer families.

Until we deal with these issues honestly, we will never create an emotional ability to deal with Alzheimer's. If we do not deal with our issues of grief around the failures of love, we cannot live with Alzheimer's disease. We are fortunate as caregivers because we get the rare opportunity to practice love every day. We step into that flow as soon as we do the smallest act of love. We can do it anytime.

It is easy to write the words but not always easy to carry out the wish and intention to be a loving caregiver. To allow an environment for love to flow, we need to take care of anything within us that stands in the way. That means becoming loving caregivers to ourselves and it especially means forgiving ourselves.

We show we have forgiven ourselves when we begin to treat ourselves with tenderness, consideration, and kindness. Love can only work in the caregiving relationship if it works within us. I have never met an angry, overwhelmed caregiver who was not as bitter and angry and mean to himself or herself as to the person being looked after.

So be attentive to what you need and make sure you get as

much of it as possible. A kind relationship with oneself is essential to create an atmosphere of loving-kindness.

This does not just happen. It has to be deliberately created, and to do so you need the following:

- time to sit still
- time to sleep
- spiritual discipline
- a plan of action
- an ordering of priorities
- a balanced schedule

All of these are important to create the world in which love can flow. We have to nurture love so that love nurtures us and so that we in turn can be nurturing caregivers to someone else.

Creating a space for nurturing love in our lives then allows us to experience the greatest gift—being able to step into the flow of unconditional love.

Chapter 11

Letting Go

It is so hard to face the day when someone we care for needs more than we can provide at home. For most caregivers, this deeply painful decision is reached only after a long struggle. This is true even when the relationship between caregiver and the person with Alzheimer's is not a good one. When the relationship has been loving and connected, it is even more harrowing to have to face the fact that care is no longer possible at home.

We all feel the loss of home as a wound. The older and more settled a person is, the greater the sense of loss. And, of course, for the spouse or child, this also represents the emotional breaking up of marriage or family, a divorce of the heart made necessary by disease. Overlying the issue of placement into long-term institutional care, which cannot be underestimated, is the shadow of the workhouse or poor farm. These fears may sound like those ancient institutions out of history, but they have a real resonance for elders whose own parents dreaded ending up in aged poverty. This is another reason why, for so many older caregivers, the idea of sending a spouse off into care represents a deep abandonment and sense of guilt.

Even for the postmodern adult child, this feeling of guilt at abandoning a parent to other care is deeply painful. Only choosing good enough care can offset these feelings and enable the family to feel that they have done their best to ensure that the person with dementia will get the necessary help and support from care professionals. Such choices need time and plenty of homework, so it is never too early to do the necessary research that helps support a good decision.

There is also another way to support this decision making and that is to do the emotional homework necessary in the process of being willing to let go of being a caregiver. This involves facing the pain and confronting the feelings of guilt and abandonment that so often go with placement. One part of facing the pain is a psychological and spiritual journey of facing oneself with complete honesty and the other is the rational process of facing the fact that total care cannot be given by one person at home.

This chapter helps to guide family members through both processes and outlines the ways in which we can identify a source of good long-term care.

Q: I'm going to keep my husband home as long as I can, but I suppose the day will come when I can't care for him. How will I find the right place for him? And how will I know when he should go into care?

A: I'm glad you're thinking ahead, even though it's probably very hard to look at putting your husband into care. However, to find the place that would be best for him requires that you do your homework in advance.

Often families avoid this, presumably in some kind of denial of its necessity. Unfortunately that leads to emergency placement in the wrong kinds of care.

While you keep your husband at home, it is vitally important you educate yourself about being a caregiver. Get to know the disease, so you don't spend time fighting the disease itself. Attend to the task of looking after yourself too. That way, you'll avoid the health and stress problems of overburdened caregivers.

Recent studies have shown that training for caregivers makes a big difference in how long they can keep their family member at home. There are also many ways of getting help in your own home. For example, Mary and Irving have a live-in student from China who gets his board and lodging and a small salary for helping with Irving ten hours a week.

Irving likes the young man and helps him learn English; Mary gets extra free time for herself and another face around the house, which is often very cheering for her.

Using this kind of help can enable you to keep your husband home longer if you wish to. On the other hand, you may need to place him in care because you are no longer able to cope or cannot afford that kind of extra help. How do you know when to do this? You need to do it when you can no longer meet your husband's needs.

A person very disabled by dementia needs twenty-four-hour care. One person cannot give around-the-clock care and should not even try. If you had to hire nurses, they would each work an eight-hour shift—that tells you how demanding professionals regard dementia. No one ever chooses placement care too soon. Be very honest about how caregiving is affecting you, your emotional well-being, and your health, and act in time to safeguard all three.

Q: I'm afraid to bring strangers into my home to look after my wife. How do I know they won't be dishonest or weird? How do I find good helpers?

A: There are many kind, capable, and loving people available for Alzheimer's care. As you say, the trick is to find them. If you feel nervous about dealing with this yourself, you can go to a reputable agency in your area and pay their fees. Ask them about their screening process; do they check applicants' references, run a criminal check, and so on?

You might follow up on some references for yourself, if you want to be assured. If there is no such agency near you, call your local senior services or Area Agency on Aging to find out if they keep lists of live-in helpers. Ask around the community, since good helpers get known.

People advertise in local newspapers, too, and if you're prepared to take the trouble to make a thorough search, you will find someone good that way, but you must take the trouble to do so. Remember, if you start feeling discouraged, you need only one good person.

Live-in care can become as innovative as you want it to be. One lawyer decided to get help for her mother with Alzheimer's. Through a church, she found a newly arrived immigrant family who needed a home and work. They were a young couple and two children of eight and ten. They spoke little English, but the lawyer's mother was losing her language skills. The family treated the mother with love and respect and looked after her well. She enjoyed being cared for by them, and they had an easier entry into their American life.

The arrangement was so successful that after three years, when the mother died, the family stayed on in her house, now renting it. It was a totally successful experiment.

Being innovative can be the best way to deal with getting that extra help. The traditional pattern for hiring live-in help is to have one person work five days straight, with relief help for the other two days. However, this care pattern is based on the needs of the physically ill or frail elderly. It is the worst way to deal with Alzheimer care. It results in caregiver burnout and poor care, although it is an issue not being dealt with by caregivers, families, or care agencies.

Another innovative care situation was that of a seventy-six-year-old woman being cared for by four live-in caregivers, all of whom received room and board and pocket money. They shared the schedule and the caregiving tasks and led their own lives as well. Each caregiver provided one or two days a week caregiving and followed her own pattern, which created a much more interesting life for the woman they looked after. She did so well with this arrangement that in a year she underwent no drop in functioning at all.

Given that nursing homes routinely charge more than three thousand dollars a month for what is often poor Alzheimer care, it would seem practical for two or three families to get together and rent a house in which the impaired family members can be looked after by live-in caregivers on a much more personal basis.

Q: My aunt has Alzheimer's and she lives in a managed care home. The monthly fee of $2,200 is covered by her pension. She has assets of about $300,000, plus a long-term care insurance policy worth about $100,000. Don't you think it would make sense to move her into a nursing home so the insurance could be used? After all, we don't know how long she'll live.

A: Choices about care should be based on what's best for the person with Alzheimer's. They should never be based on the family's desire to start carving up the sick person's personal financial assets among themselves. There is no evidence to support the choice of nursing homes for people with dementia. In fact, from ten years of observation, I see that people often decline quickly once they go into nursing home care.

Most people think that, in Alzheimer's disease, the choices are home or nursing home, but there are several alternatives between those, some of which are actually far more appropriate for the person with Alzheimer's. The main factors that lead relatives to think about placement are:

- illness or stress on the part of the main caregiver
- incontinence in the person with Alzheimer's
- unmanageable problem behaviors in the person with Alzheimer's, especially various forms of combativeness.

These factors are not inevitable. They happen to some people and might be caused by the effect of the disease on the brain. That has never been proven. What can be seen often are reactive angry responses arising out of incidents that could have been avoided by better handling on the part of caregivers. In the same way, neither is incontinence inevitable. It has been established that only about 10 percent of people with Alzheimer's are genuinely incontinent—that is, they have truly lost bowel and bladder control. The other 90 percent are incontinent only if not helped to the bathroom often enough. They have not lost control —they simply forget.

Q: Are you saying that people with Alzheimer's don't need nursing care?

A: That's pretty much what I'm saying, as long as they don't have other specific conditions that do need nursing care. Most so-called skilled nursing care is really hygiene care and bathroom help. You get that kind of help in a good small care home or adult foster home. After all, many elders live at home with a variety of illnesses for which they take medications.

In general, people with dementia do not become completely disabled, and their care needs are not really complex, so we should be looking much more carefully at why we place them in nursing homes instead of in small care homes. The main reason is ignorance on the part of caregivers and others having the control of placement.

Doctors and lawyers typically suggest nursing homes, and it seems that most of them know little about care homes and even less about the day-to-day requirements of dementia care. Because they are professionals who strongly count upon brain work, I also suspect they have a special horror of dementia, a fear that leads them to demonize Alzheimer's disease even more than the general population. This may make them feel that such care must be overwhelming enough to require major medical nursing.

Small care homes, if they are good, supply the companionship, the routine of normal life, and the comfortingly familiar structure that truly help the person with Alzheimer's. Just like nursing homes, they are licensed and inspected by the state and they have the same chances of being good, bad, indifferent, or just okay.

Q: I think it would break my mother's heart to be put in a home. How do other Alzheimer's patients cope?

A: It is not always the deprivation you may think. For some people, their own home becomes irrelevant and even distressing. They do not recognize it. They are not really able to have their old life. Home does not feel homelike anymore. It no longer supplies a sense of home to them. They may do better in an environment designed especially for people who are impaired.

There, however, comes the rub. There are extremely few places in the country right now where impaired people can really be at home. The hospital-patterned nursing home is often the least suitable environment. The hospital-like routine, the alienating clinical look of such places, the lifestyle based on nursing care— often irrelevant to the person with Alzheimer's disease—is destructive of the person. Even though such places claim to have daylong activity programs, such claims can be spurious. Often a facility has only one or two activity staff for every fifty or sixty severely impaired people.

Dementia-specific environments are now being developed that try to create a homelike atmosphere with a protected ambience. These give the residents the freedom to wander in safety, to interact with each other or not, and to be led into activities that enhance their lives.

There are also a great many small care residences—called adult foster homes in some states, home care residences in others— available across the country.

Q: I think our father needs to go into care now. Specifically, how do we know a good place when we see it?

A: It is hard to find a good place, but the following guidelines are based on years of looking at the good, the bad, and the ugly in full-care placement. Use them while doing your homework.

In general, families tend to think that paying out large sums of money takes care of buying good standards. This, alas, is untrue.

High prices do not guarantee good care. Other things that do not guarantee good care are staff with nursing degrees, fancy wallpaper, and well-written brochures. By now, you are probably wondering how you can find your way if none of these things helps you make decisions.

Start by examining the general category of care you want. So-called skilled nursing care does not mean anything in terms of Alzheimer-specific care. The phrase *skilled nursing* often refers to the kind of care a mother gives her baby, not to any high-tech training or nursing needs. Too many nursing homes are running Alzheimer detention centers, geriatric prisons where sad inmates wander up and down corridors all day.

There are, fortunately, many stringent regulations about how residents are to be treated, but some facilities pay attention to the letter and ignore the spirit of the law. A facility could pass an official inspection with no faults and still be bad for people with Alzheimer's to live in.

Unless your father has other medical conditions that demand nursing care, or is actually bedridden or unable to walk unaided, consider a small home or adult foster care, if there is no really forward-looking Alzheimer-specific care residence in your area that you can afford.

If you do need to choose a nursing home, find one that claims to offer special care of dementia patients, then visit it more than once. Be skeptical of any claims made about Alzheimer-specific care. The reason for skepticism is that hardly anyone knows what Alzheimer residents really need for their happiness and welfare. Most facilities are concerned about efficient containment of residents and much less about their real well-being.

Often, Alzheimer residents are seen as having less status and are treated as if they had indeed lost their minds. Such treatment can be subtle. Evidence of this downgrading might be that the Alzheimer's unit is tucked away out of sight and its residents are not encouraged, even with relatives, to visit together in more open areas of the nursing home.

Alzheimer residents often get less in the way of outdoor space.

Their recreation rooms are smaller, or used mainly for dining, which means that they are not truly available. Staff do not show respect to the residents.

How can you tell whether the place you think looks good actually is good? Here are some ways to test it out.

Visit in the morning and notice how people are being treated. Is anyone being scolded for incontinence? Has someone been left half-naked in the corridor while waiting for a shower? Are the staff friendly or resentful? Can you smell urine?

Go back at mealtimes. Are people being treated with respect? If they need feeding, are they being fed considerately or is the staff member virtually force-feeding them without waiting for them to set their own pace?

Notice in general the staff's attitudes. Are they loving in voice and manner to residents? Do they actually listen to what residents say? Do they make fun of them? Are they ordering residents about as if they were children?

Also inquire about their Alzheimer-specific program. Many nursing homes claim to have special care units for people with dementias when all they have is a set of doors with alarms on them. They actually offer nothing in the way of special programming for people with Alzheimer's. Ask to see the activity program schedule, which by law is supposed to be posted on the walls of the unit. Does the program include art, music, socialization, exercise, and other specific activities such as sewing or crafts?

A good program also requires the participation and support of nursing staff. An Alzheimer unit that expects its activity staff alone to run the activity program is neglecting the well-being of residents. Any program it claims to offer is spurious, since very impaired people often need one-to-one interaction at a low level of demand and response. You should be able to see some of these people getting such attention on your visits. Sit through some of the activities and ask yourself, would this add any pleasure to my life?

What about the actual quality of interaction being offered? Are people being supported to bond with each other? People living in

Alzheimer units are often very lonely, even though they are surrounded by others and get a lot of washing, dressing, and feeding attention from the staff. And, the more impaired people are, the lonelier they will be. Therefore, what really makes a difference to them is whether anyone stops long enough to have even a tiny interaction. A good program would watch out for such residents and make sure they had the attention they needed. Many programs would continue to ignore them.

Beware of programs listing bingo, reality orientation, and reminiscence, which are largely irrelevant to people with Alzheimer's. Look for a place that has a healthy allowance for wandering. And make sure that any claims to allow such freedom are true. One nursing home made the claim that they had ten lovely acres for residents to walk through in total safety, but they also had thirty-three out of thirty-six residents tied into wheelchairs. People with Alzheimer's often need to be able to walk as a stress reliever. Constant restrictions on walking cause high levels of stress. Is there a wandering path into a garden? That would be ideal. The sad fact is that prisoners in San Quentin get a larger exercise yard than most residents in Alzheimer units in this country.

The ideal ratio would be one activity staff member to eight residents. Check out activities. Are they appropriate? Are they demeaning? How many of the residents are really taking part? Are most of them just slumped in chairs? How many people seem actually to be enjoying it?

Talk to family members of other residents and ask them what they think about the place. As well as your on-site research, check out the facility with the state licensing department. The department that licenses nursing homes—which varies from state to state, so ask your local senior services—has to keep their reports on every facility available for public reference. Read recent reports. These reports also contain complaints and follow-ups. What violations have been noted and how significant do they seem to be? Are they noted as being rectified or do they recur?

These reports will give you one insight into that nursing home. You can get another by contacting the local Ombudsman office.

The federal Ombudsman program, which operates in every state, is a long-term care advocacy agency. It oversees complaints about long-term care facilities—nursing homes, adult foster homes, units big and small. The Ombudsman volunteers go into facilities and investigate complaints. Its local offices often have a good insight into the operation of local care homes. They are likely to warn you about poor ones, and they are happy to tell you which ones rarely have complaints made about them.

All of this will give you a much better idea of what is out there. Do not let the lack of top-notch places depress you. The sad fact is that there are few really good places, but you need only one. Do not be impressed by any amount of dressing-up done to the nursing home. One nursing home in the San Francisco area spent hundreds of thousands of dollars revamping the decor—into a slightly depressing light blue ambience—and had nothing left over to buy a few benches so that Alzheimer residents could sit outside on the tiny patio that was all they had for exercise and fresh air.

Q: We're thinking of adult foster care for our mother, but she'd have to share a room with another woman. Do you think lack of privacy would bother her?

A: Since I don't know your mother, I assume you're wondering if people with dementia in general are bothered by lack of privacy. Usually in foster homes, two people share bedrooms, unless a family is willing to pay a double fee to hold the whole room for one person. This sharing is not necessarily a bad thing for people with Alzheimer's. They may feel very frightened and lonely by themselves, since they tend to live in an unidentifiable, timeless place, and having another person around can be comforting. This does not mean there will not be occasional quarrels, but they are not necessarily a bad sign. People who share rooms are bound to raid each other's clothes and closets, but this is also Alzheimer normality. It may be possible to find care residences that offer individual rooms, but the rates are higher and it is not necessarily more pleasing to the patient.

Too much stimulation can be stressful for the person with dementia, but sharing a room does not usually seem to be a cause of stress. It's probably more like a college roommate situation.

You can check out care homes just as you do nursing homes. Visit and see what you think. Here are some warning signs to look for:

- television being used as an electronic babysitter
- radio tuned to a rock station
- bad smells
- improperly dressed residents, unless they have chosen this and are being respected for their choice
- cold, uncaring caregivers
- no activities and no outings. There should be regular outings every week—to a senior lunch, to an ice cream parlor, to the park, to something somewhere. Ideally, there should also be activities in the house—exercises, pet visits.

An ideal care home might have any or all of the following:
- a pleasant garden
- some pets
- planned schedule of activities
- good food
- regular staff training and little turnover of staff, though this can be an elusive goal in an industry where workers are often ill-paid. Staff should be responsive to your needs and those of your relative, not resentful of your expressing them.

The typical care home is a personal residence in which the home care part is paying for the real estate. Either the owner lives there or has a live-in manager. A good place will have the owner on site most days, since home care staff need this kind of encouragement to keep standards high.

Q: *We've found what seems like a nice place for our uncle to live, but it's run by Koreans who don't seem to speak much English. We don't know how he'll understand them. Do you think we're worrying too much?*

A: Yes. First, this is a situation that will improve anyway as the Koreans live here longer, and their children will undoubtedly help out with communication problems.

Second, good English is not nearly as important as a good heart. In the last few years, the care home business has attracted many Asian Americans, often those who are fairly new to this country. Many Asians tend to have a much more reverent and accepting attitude toward elders and a natural kindness toward them, which usually tends to overcome any small problems around language communication.

Q: *We like the idea of a small care home but our doctor says since Grandfather will have to go into a nursing home eventually, this will save trauma later. Do you agree?*

A: Absolutely not. I don't believe in giving people the worst choice now on the theory that they'll have to be there eventually. There's nothing to say your grandfather will ever need nursing care. Even if he does, are you going to deny him quality life now and for the next few years based on a future you can't predict?

It is certainly true that there is some trauma attached to any move for a person with Alzheimer's. Often a move causes a temporary loss of functioning, which may slowly improve, although it may never return to original levels. This must be a personal choice, and you may want to opt for a one-time-only choice and therefore go straight for the nursing home.

However, it is very important that we do not undervalue the pleasure of life in the moment. You may suffer to see your relative becoming more ill, but it is likely that your relative will experience a lot of happiness in the average day. The most supportive and friendly environment for the individual's functioning would always be a good direction to go in, even if it means a second move later on.

It is a sad fact that people in nursing homes often die in the weeks after admission. Some of that mortality, arguably, has to do with the shock of going into an environment that does not really support individuality.

That move might never come about. For one thing, it may be possible for your relative to stay in the home care residence until death. Local authorities can be very understanding of the need to keep someone in a familiar environment. Second, we can never predict how or when someone will die. Try not to make a decision based on some imagined future. Rather, take the situation now and ask yourself where your relative would be the happiest.

Q: What kind of environment do people with dementia need?

A: First, they need each other. Mixed populations of demented and nondemented people don't work. This is not like putting together children of mixed abilities so they can all learn from each other.

The frail, sick, and demented elderly do not have the energy to meet, exchange, and grow from each other's differences. They are angry and resentful of each other. The nondemented resident is often unkind, if not actually mean and combative, toward those who have dementia. They dislike these patients rummaging in their belongings and getting into their space. They simply can't cope with the intrusions of dementia. It is unfair to force these two different-need groups together to make each other miserable simply for a democratic principle transplanted from child care. Each type of resident needs the peace to be who they are.

Aside from that, the ideal Alzheimer environment would be bright and cheerful, with homelike bedrooms. The outdoors would include wandering paths to lead the person along and back again to some central point as well as safe access to outdoors and real freedom to wander at will in a protected environment.

There should be a high staff-to-resident ratio, and that ratio must mean actual available staff there for relationship with the resident. The therapeutic program should incorporate art, psychology, support group, and music, as well as room for family members to take part in programs, to spend time privately with the resident, and to participate in support groups.

Plenty of soft, warm places, chairs, toys, blankets, and all the same things that give children comfort should be available. The Alzheimer environment should also include normal day-to-day activities, such as helping out with carefully structured tasks, gardening, keeping pets, feeding birds, and so on. Most of all, respect for the spirit and heart of the resident must be shown by environment, treatment, and program elements.

There are few programs like this, unfortunately, but we have to hope they will increase, and soon.

Q: Is there some special way to make the transition from home into care?

A: That is a wonderful question and one that people seldom even think about. Most often they just drop their family member off at the new living space, hang around for a while, then go. Of course, if the new place is some distance away, it may be impractical to have a gradual transition. Most nursing homes have no capacity to deal with drop-in visits from prospective residents.

If possible, you might take your relative along for a friendly visit to the place you have in mind and see how that goes. It may at least help put your mind at ease. If that goes well, you will probably feel better about allowing the placement. Of course, if you are already burnt out as a caregiver, this will probably come as a welcome relief to you.

If you have close emotional attachment to your relative or spouse, you may feel sad, as if you are abandoning someone you love. You are certainly not abandoning that person—the bill alone, alas, will remind you of that—but you are buying care you can no longer supply. There is no ideal way to decide how to proceed at placement. Some people go on a brief holiday for a few days, to get a much-needed break and to let the person settle in. Reaction to placement is an individual matter, and there are no rules. Pay attention to your own intuition.

Q: We recently had to put my husband into a care home. He's become much worse since he's been there. Does this mean it was a mistake?

A: Not at all. Often people become much more obviously demented once they move into long-term care. It is as if they have the freedom finally to give way to the true extent of their illness. There is no more need to cover up. This is what we often see in the new arrival—a downturn in functioning.

Don't let this worry you. It is the shock and trauma of environmental change; most people recover from this, especially if the environment is supportive of them and they receive enough love and reassurance from staff.

You may find that your husband weeps when you visit, or he may be angry or unpleasant, even though none of this happens when you are not present. It is not a sign that your visit is disturbing or unwelcome. On the contrary, it shows you are trusted enough for real feelings to emerge; this may not always feel like a privilege, but it is. You may not always find that things are as you would want them to be, and indeed nowhere is perfect.

If you have been a really good caregiver to your spouse, you may have to accept that no one will look after him as well as you did. You must adjust to the idea that "good enough" will have to do.

Chapter 12

Approaching
the End

There's a lot of misinformation on Alzheimer's disease and death. Although you'll hear that people die of it, few actually die of Alzheimer's. But, if they do, they die easily.

Death is often seen as a release for a family living with Alzheimer's disease and, in fact, the typical Alzheimer death usually comes gently. It comes with the inward dreaming of a person already absorbed in the internal process of dying, a state resembling sleep or a turning away from consciousness. It is nothing to fear. It has no pain or fearsome aspects. It is not different from the way a child sleeps; sleep becomes deeper and consciousness weaker, until there is an end to life. This is the typical Alzheimer death.

Q: What do people with Alzheimer's actually die of? What kills them?

A: A good question, one without a reliable answer because of the nature of Alzheimer's itself. Although called a disease, it is more of a syndrome, a collection of symptoms gathered in a body and a brain failing from the center, presumably from the neurostructure of the brain itself.

Once a person has been diagnosed as having Alzheimer's disease, no matter what the actual cause of death, it is likely to be listed as Alzheimer's disease, in the same way that people with AIDS are listed as dying of AIDS when in fact they die of other specific conditions.

Some people become obsessed by pictures of what they imagine to be the real Alzheimer death—a victim lying helpless in bed, being fed (perhaps intravenously), not speaking, not moving, not responding, emaciated, needing to be diapered. This is not the usual fate of people with Alzheimer's. On the contrary, it is quite unusual. People with Alzheimer's usually die of the same things as everyone else—cancer, heart problems, lung problems.

Q: So what about the terminal stage of Alzheimer's? Does everyone go through that before they die?

A: No. In fact, it happens as rarely as about one person in thirty. Even in a special Alzheimer unit in a skilled nursing facility in the San Francisco Bay Area, only two out of fifty-four people were bedridden, even though many of the residents had been in care for several years.

Of those who died in a three-month period, none died in what many people dread is the classic Alzheimer way. Five people died within weeks of admission to the unit. Of the other deaths, one person died as a result of complications from a fall caused by the side effects of psychotropic medications; two died of cancer; two had strokes and subsequently developed pneumonia and died; one had a cold, which his family refused to have treated by antibiotics when it went into his chest. He then developed pneumonia and died. This picture of the range of deaths is quite typical.

Q: I'm so afraid my mother will end up like those people you hear about, lying in diapers and needing help with everything, just like a baby. Do you have any advice for coping with that?

A: First, don't envision such pictures in advance. You cannot possibly know what your mother's death will be like, so there is no point in worrying about it until the time comes.

In Alzheimer's, as in many other difficult situations, taking life one day at a time is the key to managing stress. Also, don't project your present fears into your mother's future. As distressing as it may feel to see someone you care about in that condition, that same consciousness is not present in that person when she reaches such a stage. In other words, we all tend to get on with whatever our daily life is—because that's mainly the only option we have.

It's amazing how little people manage with when they have to. The key in all care is how much support and kindness we get from those around us. They have the power to demean or honor us by their attitudes.

Q: *Should we do something about our mother's medical wishes if she should come to the terminal stages of Alzheimer's? She hasn't signed one of those papers yet. Is it too late? We know she wouldn't want her life prolonged unnaturally.*

A: It's good you're thinking about this before the time comes to face your mother's death. There are some major decisions to make about health care and about death.

The most difficult issue for caregivers and family members is deciding what would be appropriate and acceptable medical intervention for the impaired person. All such issues should be decided before a time of crisis, since few families can react completely rationally when face to face with an emergency.

Death is inevitable for every one of us. After we are born, it is the only other thing guaranteed. Although we know technically we are not immortal, we generally live that way until the prospect of death intervenes.

When a person is diagnosed as having Alzheimer's disease, death is sending a message that it is on its way. Therefore, as a concerned family member, you need to think through certain issues that acknowledge that message.

Most states allow people to make these major health care decisions and record them in some legal way. Some states, such as California, require families to record their wishes on paper when their relative is admitted to a care center. Since these laws vary, you need to find out what your state requires for you to make your wishes known.

I don't know how complicated it will be for you, since apparently your mother made no such declaration before diagnosis. It may take only a declaration to your doctor, or require that you sign a simple legally binding document, but in some states you may have to get an attorney to draw up health care papers, either as a living will or as a power of attorney for health care.

Your mother isn't necessarily incompetent to make such decisions for herself. Even with dementia, people can make valid and sensible choices for themselves. Much will depend on your lawyer's advice.

Q: How can we decide whether, for example, to allow our uncle to have a feeding tube if he can't feed himself anymore? Would he suffer if he wasn't fed? How can we know these things?

A: If your uncle can't feed himself, someone will feed him. However, in some cases, toward the end of life, people become unable to take any food by mouth. This seems to be basically a failure of the whole system—cognitive, neuromuscular, and emotional. It comes when life is effectively drawing to a close. Artificial intervention can be made at this point, in the form of either intravenous feeding or surgical introduction of a tube into the stomach.

This is a very personal issue that people may deeply disagree over. Even nursing staff can become very emotional about this issue. One woman who wanted her mother to have a feeding tube withdrawn was shouted at by the nursing director, "Do you really want your mother to starve to death?" Of course, she hardly felt that she could answer "Yes."

Do what seems right to you, because you will be the one living with that decision for the rest of your life. If you really feel strongly that life-prolonging measures should be taken, you must choose accordingly.

Consider the following to help you make decisions:

1. Will intervention cause extra suffering for your uncle? Do not believe anyone who tells you that feeding tubes are not uncomfortable. If you have ever had a catheter, a nose tube, or a stomach tube inserted, you know they are uncomfortable.
2. Will this intervention keep your uncle more comfortable or will it merely extend life?
3. Is life extension more important than allowing a peaceful death?
4. Are you making a decision based on what makes you comfortable or what will make your uncle comfortable?
5. Are you afraid to think about death? If so, be suspicious of your own choice for life no matter what its condition.
6. Read about death and the dying process.

Some excellent books are available, and you can also find good workshops offered locally. Ask your local hospice helpers or contact your local AIDS organization, since both work closely with the dying.

Let us assume that you have made all your medical decisions and that your uncle is dying. If no food is being taken, death will probably occur in two weeks, give or take a few days.

If you're up to it, you might visit some elders who are dying. Nothing makes as much sense as knowing from participation what the dying process is all about.

Q: I'd like to bring my mother home for her last days. Is that a silly idea?

A: I think it's a magnificent idea—provided you're fully prepared. That means practical arrangements and emotional preparedness.

You can get a great deal of help from your local medical services—nursing help, home health aides, medical devices, hospice workers—if you want to do this.

It is not easy. It is hard work, even with all that help, but for some people it can be a wonderful time of closure. Those who have done it don't regret it.

Don't feel obligated to, though. You must feel reasonably comfortable with the idea. On the other hand, don't let anyone talk you out of it if you really want to do it. Although people talk of the dying needing skilled nursing care, what they usually need is the kind of care you would give a baby.

If there are no extra medical problems—open wounds, tubes, seizures—a person dying of Alzheimer's disease needs to be kept clean, dry, watered, and warm. You will be able to learn everything you need to know in one day. I say this not to push you into such a decision, but to let you know what is realistically possible.

There are some excellent practical books about looking after the dying. They are available at public libraries. Also your local public health nurse will help you learn what you need to know about looking after your mother.

Much of what you will need is your own ability to be still with your mother. Whether someone dies at home or in some kind of care situation, the essential need of the dying is to have a human being with them for the journey. If you choose, you can make the journey to death a very special time in your relationship with your mother. It needs your patience and your presence. People who are dying, with Alzheimer's disease or not, are usually very absorbed in the inward process of their journey. It is common for them to slip in and out of sleep, even to appear to be in a coma, although at some deep level they know that you are there.

It is easy to think that is not true, but we know from many accounts of people in comas who later recover that they have a deep awareness of everything going on around them. They may not be able to do more than twitch or slightly open their eyes, but that is the only way in which they can respond. Many an unconscious person has squeezed the hand that is squeezing theirs, so never feel that someone is beyond being reached. It simply is not true.

Q: *I've heard that people with Alzheimer's sometimes become whole before they die. Is that true?*

A: I'm not sure they become whole, but I do know they often come to have more awareness at death than perhaps for months before that moment.

This dying time can be very useful as a process of reconciliation. This is the time to let go of anything unresolved and the time to give what this person needs—unconditional love and caring. One way in which some people have come to acceptance of Alzheimer's disease is to take the opportunity it gives to love the person.

One caregiver said, "Of course I wish my mother never got Alzheimer's disease. She had a hard life when she was young. When she was old, she became almost like a child again and I felt as if we were able to give her what she'd never had before. That's how I made sense of it to myself."

Part of the dying process is about not only giving to the person who is dying but also working through one's life story and making some sense of it. Those who work hard to be with someone in this process come to peace and resolution much more easily.

Alzheimer's disease is very hard on family relationships, and many people feel bitter and angry after the devastation of this disease. If you feel embittered or angry, the dying time is the time to confront all your feelings. Being with the dying person, and giving that person all you have to give in love and kindness, will benefit you in the end.

People who have avoided being with their relative at death are left for years afterward with feelings of bitterness, anger, and fear. The act of selflessly giving love can heal the person who gives it. Those who do not come to such resolution are often driven to try to find it with others. Alzheimer care programs are full of volunteers with unresolved feelings about the disease, still trying to resolve them long after the death of their family member.

Being present at someone's death reminds us that there is never a moment when love is irrelevant or unnecessary. It also helps us to feel less afraid of our own death and more able to live life more fully.

Chapter 13

Achieving a Sense of Closure

Moving on after the devastation of Alzheimer's—whether you have placed someone into full-time care or whether the one you cared for has died—requires the ability to bring closure to your journey.

Even though there were probably many times that you wished to be relieved of the daily burden, people often feel a sense of purposelessness and loss when the end comes. And yet, at the same time, relief can also be a predominant feeling. It is a little like being widowed and yet not being quite free to get on with the mourning.

Death and placement are different situations, but they create similar emotions for the caregiver. But, no matter what your situation, closure will bring a sense of completion to the past so that you may find new life.

Q: I've been living with my mother and looking after her, but I can't go on caring for her any longer. I've found a nice home, and I'm going to place her there. Now I find I'm panicking—not about her, but about me. How am I going to cope without having her to look after? That probably seems like a weird question!

A: No, I think it's a very aware question. You see that this move will relieve you yet remove some structure from your life. It's natural to feel a sudden fear. Change, even good change, always arouses fear in human beings.

You might trying leaving home for a while. It will give you a chance to reexamine your life away from the suddenly empty house. While you are away, make plans. Write down the things you would like to do, the ways in which you plan to restructure your life. Don't sit at home with all the time you need but nothing to do with that time. Put yourself back at the center of your life. Keep a journal to help you sort things out.

This is the time to grieve, too. Do not be afraid or ashamed to cry, if that is how you feel. If you mainly feel relief, accept it. It is very hard to look after another person in the way you have. Of course you feel relief.

You might find it useful to continue going to a support group, or to start to go if you have never been before. Other Alzheimer caregivers, of all people, know how hard it is to place your mother in a care residence. Those who will be facing your choice at some point can also benefit from your experience.

See your mother as often or as little as you feel is right for both of you. When you get especially lonely, you might like to spend some more time with her.

Your biggest task is likely to be that of rebuilding your life. You will probably have to make real efforts to do so, since it is likely your social life became fractured during your caregiving years. You might start in the way other people are advised to meet people: go to classes and activities that interest you, go to social events and social centers. The process of rebuilding will not be easy, but it is possible.

Q: *My wife's in the care home now and I hardly know what to do with myself. We don't have any friends now and the kids don't come by much. What do other old codgers do?*

A: If you're an old codger who can dance or walk, you'll find yourself in demand among widowed ladies! But that probably isn't what you're ready for at this point. I suspect you're still mourning the loss of your real married life.

If you have had years of living a full life with your wife, there is now a huge hole in your life. It will be hard work to start over, and sometimes you will feel more lonely with people than by yourself. This is normal. It is how everyone feels on being new on a social scene. Keep persevering. If your wife was always the one who kept your social life organized, you will have to make an effort to create a new one. Friendship does not just happen. Like any relationship, it needs careful nurturing, and you may have lost, or never had, the touch.

Read anything that will help you, and rebuild your interest in hobbies, cooking, fishing—whatever you used to like. Find more interests. Make a list of things you always said you would do one day when you had time—this is the time. Everyone needs some unfulfilled dreams to keep working on.

It sounds as if your relationship with your children needs some repair. Why not go to see your children and get to know them better? This is the time to reach out to them. Maybe they don't know how to do that to you. With your wife in care, you are likely to find you have a different kind of relationship with your children. It takes courage—or sometimes desperation—to rebuild what needs fixing. It will be worth trying, though.

Find something to do that involves helping other people and reaching out to others. Take a bus trip or cruise. You'll meet folks and it will give you practice at making friends. Get a pet.

If you're looking for an answer that's none of these things, find it for yourself. Maybe you have a long-ago dream you could still achieve.

Q: Is it wrong to want to go dancing while my husband's in a nursing home? My children encourage me to go, but it feels wrong to me.

A: Well, good for your children! You did a good job there, obviously. It's not wrong to dance. Do you think you should sit at home and do nothing now that your husband's in care? Not so. You have a life to live too, so make the most of it.

Maybe your guilty feeling is connected with the fact that dancing often leads to other things, like making friends or possibly being faced with a relationship choice. It's early to worry about that. Save the worry for when it happens to you. It may not arise as a problem.

This is a very personal issue, one that each person has to work out independently, and many people do work it out without too much trauma. It takes time and it takes understanding and respect from others.

There are many variations of dealing with this issue. Some people maintain a sexual partnership with their spouse, at least as long as feasible. The law, by the way, says you have the right to spend conjugal time with your spouse in privacy in a care home or facility. You can always bring your spouse home for visits, too. Do not let anyone try to make you feel ashamed if you would still like a sexual partnership. It is nobody's business but your own.

Some people choose to spend social time with others but not to take on a sexual involvement. Some people would like to have a sexual involvement but their children will not let them. This is an issue on which you will have to take your own stance. As an adult your choices are your own and you owe nothing to your children in that area. It is astonishing how many children turn into puritans where their parents' sexuality is concerned—but, presumably, they get that from their parents. You may have to struggle for your sexual independence, but stick with it. Do what you need to do and guard your rights and your privacy.

Q: *My husband's dead now. He died of a stroke in the hospital but he'd had Alzheimer's for nearly ten years. My problem is I feel so guilty all the time. Do you have a cure for guilt?*

A: If I did, I'd bottle it and sell it. You don't say why you feel guilty, but since you raise the question I will assume you did not treat your husband badly, or presumably your guilt would actually be well-placed remorse. So let's consider this.

It is very normal to feel anger and resentment toward someone who is sick with any disease, let alone a disease that demands as much from a caregiver as Alzheimer's does. This anger does not come from our rational mind but from our emotional center, which feels abandoned or used or just overwhelmed by this long ordeal. Therefore, because we know that the sick person has not deliberately become ill, we may feel guilty about our own anger. If you feel overwhelmed by these feelings, you might find it helpful to talk things over with a professional—a therapist, a counselor, a minister, a priest or rabbi, a social worker.

Interestingly, my experience shows that people who really did all they could are the ones who feel guilty that they didn't do even more. People who are negligent or mean-spirited caregivers seem to feel no guilt, only a keen sense of self-justification. So you can take it that your guilt represents uneasiness that you weren't totally perfect all the time.

Let yourself off that hook. Try meditation, stress management, or just reminding yourself that you don't have to be perfect.

Q: *My husband died three months ago and I still feel that he comes back sometimes to our house. Am I going crazy?*

A: No, this is a common phenomenon after the death of someone close. Many people experience it, so you are very normal in what you feel. There is nothing strange about this feeling. It has been noted in all cultures in all ages. You are not crazy.

We could argue over what the feeling means. Some people and many cultures accept this as a literal event, the spirit of the dead person returning from time to time. In an out-of-touch society, some professionals try to classify this as a delusion of some kind, but I don't. From my experience of living in many different cultures,

I know that it happens all over the world. Most people feel comforted by the presence of someone they loved, so allow yourself to accept that comfort.

Perhaps if you joined a grief group, you would find people to talk over all your experiences, not only this one. That way, you would be with others who truly understand and can support your process through grief and loss.

There are many support groups for the bereaved, and they can be a useful source of help as you go through the grieving process. Typically, spouses report that, contrary to what you might think, the loss is usually greater after about six months have passed. By then, often you are no longer getting the regular support of friends and family and there is less opportunity to talk about your partner. Also, life has settled into what can sometimes be a bleakness, especially if you have not worked on rebuilding a life for yourself. Keep on working at that.

Q: We buried my mother six months ago. She died of Alzheimer's disease and now I find myself getting panic-stricken every time I forget something. What are my chances of developing Alzheimer's?

A: Very small. There is little information to support the idea that Alzheimer's runs in families. Nevertheless, once you have lost a parent to Alzheimer's disease, you do worry. Your fears are natural and they complicate the grieving process you go through when you lose a parent.

There are two processes involved in the loss of a parent to Alzheimer's: coming to terms with the death and coming to terms with the disease. Both are necessary. The child who does not come to terms with Alzheimer's gets stuck in the past, often weighed down by bitterness, anger, and fear.

Very often, the people who become involved in Alzheimer respite programs are those who have not yet resolved their issues around the loss of a parent to Alzheimer's. The hardest thing to do is to sit down with our source of pain and be with it until we understand it and can move on. If, however, you can face the process, then working with people with Alzheimer's can indeed be a wonderful source of healing. It is much easier to accept Alzheimer's in a stranger, and working with Alzheimer's is one way of coming to a peaceful resolution.

Using your experience to help others is a healthy way to process your own journey, as long as you also do the inner work of resolution that is needed for you to come to peace. If you work on inner and outer worlds, improving both as you go along, you really will find some of the answers that troubled you so much. The question that is most useful is not "Why me?" but "What can this journey teach me?"

The path to peace and resolution is an individual one. Coming to a sense of closure and moving on must include some way of coming to quietness, of facing inner fears, anguishes, and pains, and some form of finding a lasting compassion from which one can reach out to others. If the answers contained in this book have helped you along your path, it has fulfilled its purpose.

Appendix A
Bibliography

CAREGIVING

Biracree, T. and N. *Over Fifty: The Resource Book.* New York: HarperCollins, 1991.

Davidson, Ann. *Alzheimer's: A Love Story: One Year in My Husband's Journey.* Palo Alto, Calif.: Birch Lane Press, 1997.

Gray-Davidson, Frena. *The Alzheimer's Sourcebook for Caregivers: A Practical Guide for Getting Through the Day.* 2d ed. Los Angeles: Lowell House, 1996.

Kübler-Ross, Elisabeth. *On Death and Dying.* New York: Macmillan, 1981.

Moore, Thomas. *Care of the Soul.* New York: Harper, 1992.

Newman, Diane Kaschak, and Mary Dzvrinko. *The Urinary Incontinence Sourcebook.* Los Angeles: Lowell House, 1997.

Pace, N. L., and P. V. Rabins. *The 36-Hour Day.* Baltimore: Johns Hopkins University Press, 1981.

Sogyal, Rinpoche. *The Tibetan Book of Living and Dying.* New York: Harper, 1993.

Thich Nath Hanh. *Peace Is Every Step.* Parallax Press, 1987.

DIET

Ames, Bruce, M.D., et al. "Oxidation and the Degenerative Diseases of Aging: A Review." *Nutritional Research Newsletter* 12, no. 3 (November/December 1993): 111.

Braly, James, M.D., and Laura Torbet. *Dr. Braly's Food Allergy and Nutrition Revolution.* New York: Keats Publishing, 1992.

Chatterjee, S. S., et al. "Studies on the Mechanism of Action of an Extract of Ginkgo Biloba." *NaunynSchmeiderberg's Arch Pharmacol* 320 (1982): R52.

Giller, Robert, M.D., and Kathy Matthews. *Natural Prescriptions.* New York: Carol Southern Books, 1994.

Hass, H. "Brain Disorders and Vasoactive Substances of Plant Origin." *Planta Medica Suppl.* (1981), 257–265.

Khalsa, Dharma Singh, M.D., and Cameron Stauth. *Brain Longevity: The Breakthrough Program that Improves Your Mind and Memory.* New York: Warner Books, 1997.

Kleijnen, J., et al. "Ginkgo Biloba." *Lancet* 340, no. 4 (November 7, 1992): 1136.

Koltringer, P., et al. "Mikrozirkulation und Viskoelastizitat des Vollblutes unter Ginkgo-bioloba-extrakt. Eine plazebokontrollierte, randomisierte Doppelblind–Studie." *Perfusion* 1, no. 2 (1989): 28–30.

Rai, G. S., et al. "A Double-Blind Placebo Controlled Study of Ginkgo Biloba Extract in Elderly Outpatients with Mild to Moderate Memory Impairment." *Current Medical Research Opinions* 12, no. 6 (1991): 350–55.

Russell, Robert, and Paolo Suter. "Vitamin Requirements of Elderly People." *American Journal of Clinical Nutrition* 58, no. 11 (July 1993): 4.

Vorberg, G. "Ginkgo Biloba Extract (GBE): A Longterm Study of Chronic Cerebral Insufficiency in Geriatric Patients." *Clinical Trials Journal* 22 (1985): 149–57.

"The Zinc Link to Alzheimer's: Is There a Reason to Worry?" *Environmental Nutrition* 18, no. 1 (May 7, 1995): 7.

DRUG INFORMATION

Graedon, Joe and Theresa. *50+ The People's Pharmacy for Older Adults.* New York: Bantam, 1988.

Griffith, H. W. *Complete Guide to Prescription and Non-Prescription Drugs.* New York: Berkley, 1995.

ALTERNATIVE HEALING

Homeopathy

Boericke, W., M.D. *Homeopathic Materia Medica.* Boericke, 1995.

Souter, Keith, M.D. *Homeopathy for the Third Age.* U.K.: Daniel, Saffron Waldon, 1993.

Weiner, M., Ph.D. *The Complete Book of Homeopathy.* New York: Avery, 1989.

Aromatherapy

Berwick, Ann. *Aromatherapy.* St. Paul, Minn.: Llewellyn, 1997.

Worwood, V. *The Complete Book of Essential Oils and Aromatherapy.* San Rafael, Calif.: New World Library, 1991.

Herbology

Chevallier, A. *The Encyclopedia of Medicinal Plants.* New York: Dorling Kindersley, 1997.

Ody, P. *The Complete Medicinal Herbal.* New York: Dorling Kindersley, 1993.

MEDICAID

Budish, A. *Beating the Medicaid Trap.* New York: Holt, 1994.

Inlander and Mackay. *Medicare Made Easy.* People's Medical Society, 1995.

Appendix B

Resources

ALZHEIMER'S ASSOCIATION

919 North Michigan Avenue
Chicago, IL 60611-1676
1-800-272-3900 (national toll-free number)
1-800-621-0379 (Illinois residents only)

This is the major national resource for basic information on Alzheimer's disease.

TOLL-FREE HELPLINES

Senior Helpline, 1-800-328-7576 (at Brigham Young University), offers more than 100 recorded tapes of help to elders.

National Institute on Adult Day Care, 1-800-424-9046, can refer you to the nearest adult day care center.

American Health Assistance Foundation, 1-800-437-2423, provides education materials on Alzheimer's relief programs and provides funding, including financial assistance to families in need of relief services.

SOURCES FOR SUPPLIES

Homeopathy

Although your local health food store or holistic healing store will probably carry remedies, these are additional resources for homeopathic remedies.

Homeopathic Educational Services
2124 Kittredge St., Berkeley, CA 94704
(Remedies, tapes, kits, books. Send SASE for catalog.)

National Center for Homeopathy
801 North Fairfax St., Suite 306, Alexandria, VA 22314.
(703) 548-7790
(They can supply a list of homeopaths in your area.)

International Foundation for Homeopathy
23600 Eastlake Ave. E., #301, Seattle, WA 98102
(206) 324-8230
(They can also supply a list of homeopaths in your area if you
    phone or write.)

Aromatherapy
All the following will send a catalog of supplies if you send a SASE:

Essentially Yours North America
P.O. Box 81866, Bakersfield, CA 93380

Aroma Vera
P.O. Box 3609, Culver City, CA 90231

Original Swiss Aromatics
P.O. Box 606, San Rafael, CA 94915

Appendix C
Agency on Aging

The Agency on Aging has branches in every state and most local areas. Their task is to oversee, coordinate, initiate, and support special services for elders. Usually, you will find a local listing under "Agency on Aging" in your telephone book. If you don't, there will be state listings in your state capital. Call that number to get in touch with your local resources. If directory assistance cannot help you get that number, call the national hotline of the National Council on the Aging at 1-800-424-9046.

State Agencies on Aging

ALABAMA
Region IV
Martha Murphy Beck, Executive Director
Alabama Commission on Aging
RSA Plaza, Suite 470
770 Washington Avenue
Montgomery, AL 36130
(334) 242-5743 • FAX: (334) 242-5594

ALASKA
Region X
Connie Sipe, Director
Alaska Commission on Aging
Division of Senior Services
Department of Administration
3601 C Street, #310
Juneau, AK 99503
(907) 563-5654 • FAX: (907) 562-3040

ARIZONA
Region IX
Henry Blanco, Acting Administrator
Aging and Adult Administration
Department of Economic Security
1789 West Jefferson, 950A Street
Phoenix, AZ 85007
(602) 542-4446 • FAX: (602) 542-6575

ARKANSAS
Region VI
Herb Sanderson, Director
Division Aging and Adult Services
Arkansas Dept. of Human Services
P.O. Box 1437, Slot 1412
1417 Donaghey Plaza South
Little Rock, AR 72203-1437
(501) 682-2441 • FAX: (501) 682-8155

CALIFORNIA
Region IX
Dixon Arnette, Director
California Department of Aging
1600 K Street
Sacramento, CA 95814
(916) 322-5290 • FAX: (916) 324-1903

COLORADO
Region VIII
Rita Barreras, Manager
Aging and Adult Services
Department of Social Services
110-16th Street, Suite 200
Denver, CO 80202-5202
(303) 620-4147 • FAX: (303) 620-4189

CONNECTICUT
Region I
Christine M. Lewis, Director
Community Services
Division of Elderly Services
25 Sigourney Street
Hartford, CT 06106-5033
(203) 424-5281 • FAX: (203) 424-4952

DELAWARE
Region III
Eleanor Cain, Director
Delaware Department of Health and Social Services
Division of Services for Aging and Adults with Physical Disabilities
1901 North DuPont Highway
New Castle, DE 19720
(302) 577-4791 • FAX: (302) 577-4793

DISTRICT OF COLUMBIA
Region III
Jearline Williams, Executive Director
District of Columbia Office on Aging
441 Fourth Street, N.W., Suite 900 South
Washington, DC 20001
(202) 724-5622 • FAX: (202) 724-4979

FLORIDA
Region IV
Bentley Lipscomb, Secretary
Department of Elder Affairs
4040 Esplanade Way
Tallahassee, FL 32399-7000
(904) 414-2000 • FAX: (904) 414-6216

GEORGIA
Region IV
Judy Hagebak, Director
Division of Aging Services
Department of Human Resources
2 Peachtree Street N.E., 18th Floor
Atlanta, GA 30303
(404) 657-5258 • FAX: (404) 657-5285

GUAM
Region IX
Arthur U. San Agustin, MHR, Acting Administrator
Division of Senior Citizens
Department of Public Health and Social Services
P.O. Box 2816
Agana, Guam 96932
(671) 475-0262/3 • FAX: (671) 477-2930

HAWAII
Region IX
Marilyn Seely, Director
Hawaii Executive Office on Aging
335 Merchant Street, Room 241
Honolulu, HI 96813
(808) 586-0100   •   FAX: (808) 586-0185, modem 586-0184

IDAHO
Region X
Jesse Berain, Director
Idaho Commission on Aging
Room 108, Statehouse
Boise, ID 83720
(208) 334-3833   •   FAX: (208) 334-3033

ILLINOIS
Region V
Maralee Lindley, Director
Illinois Department on Aging
421 East Capitol Avenue, Suite 100
Springfield, IL 62701-1789
(217) 785-2870
Chicago Office: (312) 814-2630   •   FAX: (217) 785-4477

INDIANA
Region V
Bobby Conner, Director
Division of Disability, Aging and Rehabilitative Services
Family and Social Services Administration
Bureau of Aging and In-Home Services
402 W. Washington Street
Indianapolis, IN 46207-7083
(317) 232-1147   •   FAX: (317) 232-7867

IOWA
Region VII
Betty Grandquist, Executive Director
Department of Elder Affairs
Jewett Building, Suite 236
914 Grand Avenue
Des Moines, IA 50319
(515) 281-4646   •   FAX: (515) 281-4036

KANSAS
Region VII
Thelma Hunter Gordon, Secretary
Department on Aging
Docking State Office Building, Room 150
915 S.W. Harrison
Topeka, KS 66612-1505
(913) 296-0256 • FAX: (913) 296-0256

KENTUCKY
Region IV
S. Jack Williams, Director
Kentucky Division of Aging Services
Department for Social Services
275 East Main Street, 6 West
Frankfort, KY 40621
(502) 564-6930 • FAX: (502) 564-4595

LOUISIANA
Region VI
Robert Fontenot, Executive Director
Governor's Office of Elderly Affairs
P.O. Box 80374
Baton Rouge, LA 70898-0374
(504) 925-1700 • FAX: (504) 925-1749

MAINE
Region I
Christine Gianopoulos, Director
Bureau of Elder and Adult Services
Department of Human Services
35 Anthony Avenue
State House, Station #11
Augusta, ME 04333
(207) 626-5335 • FAX: (207) 624-5361

MARYLAND
Region III
Sue Ward, Director
Maryland Office on Aging
State Office Building, Room 1004
301 West Preston Street
Baltimore, MD 21201-2374
(410) 225-1102 • FAX: (410) 333-7943

MASSACHUSETTS
Region I
Franklin Ollivierre, Secretary
Massachusetts Executive Office of Elder Affairs
One Ashburton Place, 5th Floor
Boston, MA 02108
(617) 727-7750 • FAX: (617) 727-9368

MICHIGAN
Region V
Diane K. Braunstein, Director
Office of Services to the Aging
P.O. Box 30026
Lansing, MI 48909
(517) 373-8230 • FAX: (517) 373-4092
Director: (517) 373-7876

MINNESOTA
Region V
James G. Varpness, Executive Secretary
Minnesota Board on Aging
444 Lafayette Road
St. Paul, MN 55155-3843
(612) 296-2770 • FAX: (612) 297-7855

MISSISSIPPI
Region IV
Eddie Anderson, Director
Division of Aging and Adult Services
750 State Street
Jackson, MS 39202
(601) 359-4925 • FAX: (601) 359-4370

MISSOURI
Region VII
Jerry Simon, Acting Director
Division on Aging
Department of Social Services
P.O. Box 1337
615 Howerton Court
Jefferson City, MO 65102-1337
(314) 751-3082 • FAX: (314) 751-8493

MONTANA
Region VIII
Charles Rehbein, Aging Coordinator
Senior and Long Term Care Division
Department of Public Health and Human Services
P.O. Box 4210
Helena, MT 59604
(406) 444-5900 • FAX: (406) 444-7788

NEBRASKA
Region VII
Mark Intermil, Director
Department of Health and Human Services
Division on Aging
P.O. Box 95044
301 Centennial Mall South
Lincoln, NE 68509-5044
(402) 471-2306 • FAX: (402) 471-4619

NEVADA
Region IX
Carla Sloane, Administrator
Nevada Division for Aging Services
Department of Human Resources
340 North 11th Street, Suite 203
Las Vegas, NV 89101
(702) 486-3545 • FAX: (702) 486-3572

NEW HAMPSHIRE
Region I
Ronald Adcock, Director
Division of Elderly and Adult Services
State Office Park South
115 Pleasant Street, Annex Building #1
Concord, NH 03301-6501
(603) 271-4680 • FAX: (603) 271-4643

NEW JERSEY
Region II
Ruth Reader, Assistant Commissioner
Department of Health and Senior Services
Division of Senior Affairs
101 South Broad Street, CN 807
Trenton, NJ 08625-0807
1-800-792-8820
(609) 292-3766 • FAX: (609) 633-6609

NEW MEXICO
Region VI
Michelle Lujan Grisham, Director
State Agency on Aging
La Villa Rivera Building, Ground Floor
228 East Palace Avenue
Santa Fe, NM 87501
(505) 827-7640 • FAX: (505) 827-7649

NEW YORK
Region II
Walter G. Hoefer, Executive Director
New York State Office for the Aging
2 Empire State Plaza
Albany, NY 12223-1251
1-800-342-9871
(518) 474-5731 • FAX: (518) 474-0608

NORTH CAROLINA
Region I
Bonnie Cramer, Director
Division of Aging
CB 29531
693 Palmer Drive
Raleigh, NC 27626-0531
(919) 733-3983 • FAX: (919) 733-0443

NORTH DAKOTA
Region VII
Linda Wright, Director
Department of Human Services
Aging Services Division
600 South 2nd Street, Suite 1C
Bismarck, ND 58504
(701) 328-2577 • FAX: (701) 328-5466

NORTH MARIANA ISLANDS
Region IX
Gregorio S. Delos Reyes, Administrator
Office on Aging
Department of Community and Cultural Affairs
Civic Center
Commonwealth of the Northern Mariana Islands
Saipan, MP 96950
9-10-288-011-670-234-6011
FAX: 9-10-288-011-670-234-2565

OHIO
Region V
Judith V. Brachman, Director
Ohio Department of Aging
50 West Broad Street, 8th Floor
Columbus, OH 43266-0501
(614) 466-5500 • FAX: (614) 466-5741

OKLAHOMA
Region VI
Roy R. Keen, Division Administrator
Services for the Aging
Department of Human Services
P.O. Box 25352
Oklahoma City, OK 73125
(405) 521-2281 or 521-2327 • FAX: (405) 521-2086

OREGON
Region X
James C. Wilson, Administrator
Senior and Disabled Services Division
500 Summer Street, N.E., 2nd Floor
Salem, OR 97310-1015
(503) 945-5811 • FAX: (503) 373-7823

PALAU
Region X
Lillian Nakamura, Director
State Agency on Aging
Republic of Palau
Koror, PW 96940
9-10-288-011-680-488-2736
FAX: 9-10-288-680-488-1662 or 1597

PENNSYLVANIA
Region III
Richard Browdie, Secretary
Pennsylvania Department of Aging
Commonwealth of Pennsylvania
400 Market Street, 6th Floor
Harrisburg, PA 17101-2301
(717) 783-1550 • FAX: (717) 772-3382

PUERTO RICO
Region II
Ruby Rodriguez Ramirez, M.H.S.A., Executive Director
Commonwealth of Puerto Rico
Governor's Office of Elderly Affairs
Call Box 50063
Old San Juan Station, PR 00902
(809) 721-5710, 721-4560, 721-6121 • FAX: (809) 721-6510

RHODE ISLAND
Region I
Barbara Casey Ruffino, Director
Department of Elderly Affairs
160 Pine Street
Providence, RI 02903-3708
(401) 277-2858 • FAX: (401) 277-3664

AMERICAN SAMOA
Region IX
Lualemaga E. Faoa, Acting Director
Agency on Aging and Food and Nutrition Services (AAFNS)
Government of American Samoa
Pago Pago, American Samoa 96799
9-10-288-011-684-633-1251 or 633-7720
FAX: 9-10-288-011-684-633-2533 or 633-7723

SOUTH CAROLINA
Region IV
Constance C. Rinehart, Executive Director
South Carolina Division on Aging
202 Arbor Lake Drive, Suite 301
Columbia, SC 29223-4535
(803) 737-7500 • FAX: (803) 737-7501

SOUTH DAKOTA
Region VIII
Gail Ferris, Administrator
Office of Adult Services and Aging
Richard F. Kneip Building
700 Governors Drive
Pierre, SD 57501-2291
(605) 773-3656 • FAX: (605) 773-6843

TENNESSEE
Region IV
Emily Wiseman, Executive Director
Commission on Aging
Andrew Jackson Building, 9th Floor
500 Deaderick Street
Nashville, TN 37243-0860
(615) 741-2056 • FAX: (615) 741-3309

TEXAS
Region VI
Mary Sapp, Executive Director
Texas Department on Aging
P.O. Box 12786 Capitol Station
Austin, TX 78711
(512) 444-2727 • FAX: (512) 440-5290

UTAH
Region VIII
Helen Goddard
Division of Aging and Adult Services
P.O. Box 45500
120 North 200 West
Salt Lake City, UT 84145-0500
(801) 538-3910 • FAX: (801) 534-4395

VERMONT
Region I
Lawrence G. Crist, Commissioner
Vermont Department of Aging and Disabilities
Waterbury Complex
103 South Main Street
Waterbury, VT 05676
(802) 241-2400 • FAX: (802) 241-2325

VIRGINIA
Region III
Thelma Bland, Commissioner
Virginia Department for the Aging
700 East Franklin Street, 10th Floor
Richmond, VA 23219-2327
(804) 225-2271 • FAX: (804) 371-8381

VIRGIN ISLANDS (U.S.)
Region II
Juel C. Rhymer Molloy, Commissioner
Virgin Islands Department of Human Services
Knud Hansen Complex, Building A
1303 Hospital Ground
Charlotte Amalie, VI 00840
(212) 264-2976

WASHINGTON
Region X
Charles Reed, Assistant Secretary
Aging and Adult Services Administration
Department of Social and Health Services
P.O. Box 45050
Olympia, WA 98504-5050
(360) 493-2500 • FAX: (360) 438-8633

WEST VIRGINIA
Region III
William E. Lytton, Jr., Interim Executive Director
West Virginia Commission on Aging
Holly Grove, State Capitol
1900 Kanawha Boulevard East
Charleston, WV 25305-0160
(304) 558-3317 • FAX: (304) 558-0004

WISCONSIN
Region V
Donna McDowell, Director
Bureau of Aging and Long Term Care Resources
Department of Health and Family Services
P.O. Box 7851
Madison, WI 53707
(608) 266-2536 • FAX: (608) 267-3203

WYOMING
Region VIII
Deborah Fleming, Administrator
Division on Aging
Department of Health
117 Hathaway Building, Room 139
Cheyenne, WY 82002-0480
(307) 777-7986 • FAX: (307) 777-5340

Index

About the Author

Frena Gray-Davidson is a self-described "Alzheimer's foot-soldier" and an Alzheimer's educator. She learned almost everything she knows about Alzheimer's care from people with dementia.

Gray-Davidson has worked as a medical social worker for an Alzheimer's care unit in the San Francisco area, and she set up respite programs, including one that is part of the national model Alzheimer's respite care center. She has been a support group facilitator for the Alzheimer's Association; was the manager of a dementia-only care home in Portland, Oregon; and worked as a journalist in Asia for fifteen years. She is also the author of twelve other books of fiction and nonfiction. Gray-Davidson gives Alzheimer's workshops and training sessions nationally and internationally for family members and health professionals.

Readers may contact her via the nonprofit Alzheimer's education organization, SHACTI, at P.O. Box 361, Yachats, OR 97498, U.S.A., (541) 547-3140, or by e-mail: frgrayda@orednet.org. You can also visit her Web page at: http://www.geocities.com/HotSprings/1159.